TELEPATHY AND CLAIRVOYANCE

Founded by C. K. Ogden

The International Library of Psychology

GENERAL PSYCHOLOGY
In 38 Volumes

TELEPATHY AND CLAIRVOYANCE

RUDOLF TISCHNER

Introduction by E J Dingwall

First published in 1925 by
Routledge, Trench, Trubner & Co., Ltd.

Reprinted in 1999 by
Routledge
2 Park Square, Milton Park, Abingdon, Oxon, OX14 4RN

Transferred to Digital Printing 2007

Routledge is an imprint of the Taylor & Francis Group

© 1925 Rudolf Tischner, Translated by W D Hutchinson

British Library Cataloguing in Publication Data
A CIP catalogue record for this book
is available from the British Library

Telepathy and Clairvoyance
ISBN 0415-21045-3
General Psychology: 38 Volumes
ISBN 0415-21129-8
The International Library of Psychology: 204 Volumes
ISBN 0415-19132-7

Printed and bound by CPI Antony Rowe, Eastbourne

INTRODUCTION

THE subject matter of this volume is probably more familiar to English-speaking people than to students on the Continent. Through the work of the Society for Psychical Research in England a mass of fully documented material has been collected and partly published, whilst in the United States the labours of Dr. J. H. Hyslop, formerly Professor of Logic and Ethics, Columbia University, New York, resulted in a similar discussion of the same phenomena and the publication of selected cases. Dr. Tischner has devoted himself primarily to a consideration of certain obscure mental phenomena, which he groups into two main classes, naming them respectively *Telepathie* (telepathy) and *Hellsehen* (clairvoyance). By telepathy he means, roughly speaking, what Myers defined as " the communication of impressions of any kind from one mind to another, independently of the recognized channels of sense ". On the other hand, by the term clairvoyance he includes practically all those mental phenomena which form the basis of the researches undertaken by students of this field of inquiry.

Telepathy itself was unknown as a demonstrable fact before 1882, when the classic series of experiments with the Misses Creery were conducted by Sir William Barrett, Professor Henry Sidgwick, Mr. F. W. H. Myers, and Mr. Edmund Gurney. Since those days the Society has published a great number of cases, both those in which the faculty appeared spontaneously and also those where experimental methods were employed. In clairvoyance of the kind described by Dr. Tischner the apparent paucity of suitable subjects has made exhaustive examination of these occurrences impossible both in England and in America. The recent work of Dr. Gustav Pagenstecher on psychometric experiments in Mexico (*Proceedings of the American Society for Psychical Research*, January, 1922, xvi, 1) constitute a document of great importance, and although far more striking and impressive than those recorded by Dr. Tischner, probably belong to the same class, and can be considered in connexion with them. The phenomena described by the author of the following pages, together with the vast field of trance communications, constitute the bulk of what have been broadly termed the mental phenomena which are sharply divided from the other great division of psychical research, namely the physical phenomena.

There is at the present time a gradual movement amongst scientific men towards a cautious survey of the field covered by psychical research. The psychologist sees a new aspect of the mind when he considers the phenomenon of the trance, the " control " or the veridical vision. The physicist asks himself whether light may not conceivably be thrown upon the more obscure problems of matter and electrical energy if some attention be paid to such occurrences as the luminous phenomena of mediumship or the unexplained variations of temperature of the séance room. The biologist also is privately curious as to the possible bearing that teleplastic mediumship may have on the problems of life, whilst the philosopher is vaguely disturbed at the intrusion of these subjects into a domain hitherto abandoned for the most part to speculation untinged by empiricism.

It is not unreasonable to suppose that official science will eventually accept the facts here discussed and attempt to bring them into relation with other phenomena which are better understood and which require less intimate knowledge of the submerged depths of human personality. The refusal to inquire into these occurrences will break down when it is seen that far from contradicting or invalidating facts already acquired they merely supplement and enrich what has already found a secure place in the edifice of science. The difficulty of accepting such facts on the ground of possible fraud on the part of the subject may seem at first sight to be more weighty than is really the case. Human testimony being what it is, the most rigid precautions must always be taken to exclude those numberless and unsuspected sources of error which abound in such a study as this. Moreover, the selection of the observers and the experimenters must be judicious and calculated to further not only the claims of correct procedure but also the success of the experiments themselves. For the phenomena are almost unique amongst those which form the subjects of scientific inquiry. The human factor is a predominating feature and to treat mediums as machines or, like the spiritualists, as curious exhibits, is to court disaster at the outset of investigation. In order to obtain the best results the co-operation of the medium is desirable, an arrangement which in no way hinders the most exact observations. Similarly the co-operation of the " control " is to be sought, which does not in the least impose upon the investigator the necessity of accepting the claims of personality made by that intelligence. How far Dr. Tischner has succeeded in eliminating error and in selecting his witnesses will be seen from his own account of the experiments. The records he here presents must not be taken as isolated instances of unique phenomena, but merely as a representative selection of cases which have come under his own observation. Similar occurrences have been, and are still being, reported from all parts of the world. Although the value of these reports must necessarily vary, the general tenor of their contents is invariably the same. It is that under suitable conditions certain persons display faculties described by Dr. Tischner in the title of his book. However vague, transient, and difficult of voluntary execution these phenomena may be, the author is of the opinion that it is the duty of men of science to consider them seriously and to criticize them in the same spirit. For it must be remembered that serious attacks on the validity and authenticity of these occurrences are not common. Such explanations as unconscious whispering (Hansen and Lehmann) or chance coincidence are clearly untenable in a great number of cases. Dr. Tischner is wise in not attempting to detail any elaborate theories to describe the phenomena with which he deals. The volume is mainly a collection of facts, facts which await consideration and long and painstaking investigation. It was with this aim in view that the author originally presented the results of his studies to the reading public ; and it is worth recording that Professor Hans Driesch, whose *Science and Philosophy of the Organism* is well known to all students of Biology in this country, has written of it (*Badische Landeszeitung*, 1921, No. 321) :—

" Dr. Tischner's book is the best experimental work we have on this subject. We can put it side by side with the now classical reports of the Societies for Psychical Research on automatic mediumship, though these, as is well known, were concerned with a different group of supernormal phenomena."

It is to be hoped that in the present edition the English-speaking peoples may be able to link up Dr. Tischner's results with those made familiar to them by workers nearer home.

E. J. Dingwall.

London, 1924.

CONTENTS

PREFACE

THIS book is not simply a translation of the second edition (1921) of my study *Ueber Hellsehen und Telepathie*. It contains many changes and additions, as well as the records of a few more experiments. I have included a more complete survey of the German literature on the subject, thinking that it might be of use to English readers who cannot easily consult the originals.

My chief aim in the work has been to prove to some who still hesitate to accept them the reality of telepathy and clairvoyance by a series of new researches. I have added some introductory and theoretical matter, by way of explanation, to the bare experimental records, so as to make a well-rounded whole of a somewhat specialized treatise ; and the result may be regarded as a kind of introduction to parapsychology from one definite point of view. This book was written not only for philosophers and medical men, but also for students of the " occult " who may be interested in this rather unusual collection of facts. I have therefore not made any allusions to psycho-pathology, as it seems to me to be of secondary importance in this case.

I should like to thank the translator for the great care he has taken with the work.

R. TISCHNER.

MUNICH.
September, 1924.

I

INTRODUCTORY

A. Nomenclature. Prejudices and Difficulties. The Importance of the Subject

THE American philosopher William James tells us of a leading biologist who said that scientists do not recognize telepathy, "because they think that, even if such a thing were true, they ought to band together tokeep it suppressed and concealed. It would undo the uniformity of Nature and all sorts of other things without which scientists cannot carry on their pursuits." [1]

I do not know whether a Society for the Suppression of Telepathy has yet been founded, but the way in which the general public regard it has much the same result.[2] It would seem rather hopeless to write on this subject if there were not the ground for believing that everybody may not be so prejudiced and that there are many who may be led to regard the facts in a different light in the face of new *experimental facts*. The attempt is at any rate worth making.

First a few words on the meaning of the terms " telepathy " and " clairvoyance ", as these vary.

---

[1] *The Will to Believe*, p. 10.

[2] Dr. Kispert writes in *Das Weltbild ein Schwingungserzeugnis der Gehirnrinde* (Munich, 1920) : " We must reject this clairvoyance which is supposed to occur, as it is only possible to give a semblance of clairvoyance when you have previous knowledge of the facts. The man who has no previous knowledge of the facts has no clairvoyant faculty "—a truly dogmatic *petitio principii* worthy of one of the old scholastics.

I

TELEPATHY AND CLAIRVOYANCE

By *telepathy* I mean the transference of precepts, concepts, etc., from one person to another without the intervention of our normally recognized senses. I include messages transmitted intentionally or unintentionally by the conscious as well as by the subconscious mind, and use the expression " thought-transference " in the same sense.

Clairvoyance is for me a perception of events, objects, etc., which does not come through the channel of our normally recognized senses, and which is gained regardless of whether an object is near at hand (though not visible) or far away, and regardless of the distance of events in both space and time.[1] I use it in a very broad sense, including—if I do not give certain occult facts a spiritualistic interpretation—all the occult intellectual phenomena which do not come under the heading of telepathy.

I divide it into three subdivisions :—

1. *Cryptoscopy* (Bonaventura),[2] the vision of normally invisible, hidden objects near at hand, e.g. the contents of closed letters, impervious to normal sight, objects in boxes.

2. *Clairvoyance in Space*, the knowledge of events going on at a distance out of range of the normal senses at the time, so that the knowledge must have been obtained supernormally.

3. *Clairvoyance in Time*, vision into the past or future.

---

[1] Hopp made a mistake when he translated Grasset's definition of clairvoyance (*Ueber Hellsehen*, Dissertation, Königsberg, 1916, p. 12) as : " The faculty of seeing through invisible bodies." It should be " opaque " not " invisible ".

[2] This word is to be found in use in the 'fifties. It occurs in *Mysterien des Schlafes und Magnetismus* (Weimar, 1856) by Dr. Isidor Bonaventura. I have been unable to obtain a copy of the French book he quotes from, and cannot tell whether the term is used there. Dr. W. von Wasielewski first reintroduced it in this sense (Tischner : *Geschichte der Okkultistischen Forschung*, Pfullingen).

INTRODUCTORY

These different kinds of clairvoyance appear in varying forms and mixtures in different mediums. Various names have been introduced for them ("psychometry," "lucidity," etc.), but we must have some common name which will cover the whole ground ; the commonly used word " clairvoyance " seems to me to be very suitable for this purpose.

I may add here a few remarks on the word " occultism " and on terminology in general. Some people will object to its being used in this connexion, but I propose to use it till a better one turns up.

It can of course be interpreted mystically, but it need not necessarily be so. " Occult " means hidden, and it can truly be said that the phenomena we are dealing with are not commonplace. Looked at in this way the word " occult " is fairly suitable ; but let us use it merely as a denomination, like many names used in science. In medicine we have numbers of words whose popular meaning has little or nothing to do with their medical meaning, e.g. Cataract, Rheumatism, etc., and some of them even have a mystic tendency like *os sacrum* for rump-bone. So I shall use it as a comprehensive term to include this whole province, especially as it is already used in this sense in Germany.[1] I do not find the words " meta-psychic " and " parapsychic ", which have also been proposed as general terms, suitable, as they both require the assumption of too much theory ; this should be avoided in the choice of a name. " Teleplastic " and "telekinetic" are taken at their facial value—two purely physical terms—and that apart from any theoretical considerations. So I shall use the terms " para-psychical " and " paraphysical " for the psychical and physical in occult phenomena. Spiritualism, which

---

[1] The term " occultism " may also stand in English as it is sometimes used in this sense. [*Trans.*]

3

TELEPATHY AND CLAIRVOYANCE

I regard as a still questionable interpretation of occult phenomena, but which I cannot reject with a sarcastic remark, as is so often done, I shall call the "metapsychical". It is a scientific problem which requires very serious consideration.[1] I use the word "medium" without any mystical colouration. We cannot alter the fact that unfortunately we still require intermediate persons with these qualities to be able to study this field of science. The word "supernormal" I often use in the sense of "occult" to distinguish the phenomena due to telepathy and clairvoyance (supersensual insight) from those due to the action of our normal senses.

I should like to add a few remarks on so-called "thought-reading"[2] to prevent any misunderstanding. It should not be mixed up in any way with telepathy or thought-transference, but should be considered as an independent fact, it should more appropriately be called "muscle-reading". It is used to denote the faculty of certain people to carry out actions which they have been willed to carry out, or to find things which have been hidden when they hold the hand of a person who knows what they have been willed to do, or are otherwise in actual bodily contact with them. Slight contractions of the muscles, alterations of the pulse and breath, as the person accompanying the thought-reader sees him go right or wrong, and relaxes or has small inhibitory movements accordingly, are

[1] Various recent philosophers may be cited, especially Driesch's *Wirklichkeitslehre*, Leipzig, 1917.

[2] It should perhaps be stated that the English term "thought-reading" (Gedankenlesen) has not the same narrow significance as the German word. "Thought-reading" in English is a broad popular term which comprises telepathy, thought-transference, muscle-reading, stage "telepathy" and similar phenomena, all of which are confused in the popular mind. The "muscle-reading" mentioned by the author is the so-called "Cumberlandism", from Stuart Cumberland the muscle reader, who describes his effects in his books *A Thought Reader's Thoughts* (London, 1888) ; *People I have Read* (London, 1905), etc. [*Trans.*]

the decisive factors. Cases in which two persons walk side by side without actual contact are much more difficult to test ; but as a rule, here too the indications are not supernormal, and the necessary information is gained by " muscle-reading ", by the observation of the free or hesitating gait or the breath of the person accompanying the reader, or from his glances or those of the spectators ; this information being carefully combined and acted on. This is not at all easy to prove in the actual instances under observation : the easier and more reliable proof is indirect. Suppose, for instance, that the thought-reader is to take a pencil out of the waistcoat pocket of the gentleman with the red tie. It would be much simpler and more conclusive to sit beside the thought-reader and transmit to him telepathically the words " gentleman ", " red ", " tie ", " pencil ", or any other definite concept, if the latter really gets his information supernormally. But most " thought-readers " fail signally in this type of experiment, whereas they are very successful in the ordinary way. The only conclusion we can come to is that this difference in the possibility of solution must be due to a difference in the objects in view and their peculiarities. The real difference between successful and unsuccessful experiments is that in the former the problems to be solved consist solely of movements. This is probably where the flaw arises. Movements of some kind may occur which the thought-reader can perceive normally. Of course, a true telepathic medium will be able to solve this kind of problem as well, but we must eliminate this possibility of error to prove true telepathy.

The scientific discoverers of muscle-reading poured out the baby with the bath. They showed that muscle-reading was the true cause of this kind of thought-reading, and supposed themselves to have thereby proved that telepathy did not exist. W. Preyer,[1] a well-known physiologist, thought that he had succeeded in solving this question when he published a somewhat superficial discourse showing only a moderate degree of knowledge and based on a rather shallow study of the subject. It is quite clear that given proper experimental conditions, for instance, experiments where no motions were to be carried out, it would be quite impossible to read the simplest thought by muscle-reading. But as thought-transference was not unknown when he wrote, he should at least have gone into the matter seriously, he could not have failed to realize that his explanation did not cover all the facts. As it is, the bias against telepathy has only been strengthened by a statement of this kind from a scientist of his standing.

Some years ago, telepathy and clairvoyance were fully recognized facts. Philosophers like Hegel, Schelling, Schopenhauer, T. H. Fichte, von Hartmann, and a number of prominent medical men spoke of them as accepted facts. It is only in the last decades that this whole field of study has been looked upon as non-existent, at any rate in Germany. Science turned to other spheres of activity and dropped the whole of this region out of its interests. The proof that such a thing as clairvoyance or telepathy did not or could not exist was never brought forward; it was ignored; and that not because a close acquaintance with it seemed unworthy of study, but because it was not known. So we must put the question afresh, in a way which will adapt it to the present time and make it accessible to the methods used in modern psychology. It is only by exact experimentation that we can draw attention to it and give it its previous standing. This is where the main difficulty lies; it is rarely possible to produce the phenomena at will; they mostly come

[1] *Die Erklärung des Gedankenlesens*, Leipzig, 1886.

spontaneously and quite unexpectedly. Also, the faculty of producing them seems to dwindle for longer or for shorter periods without any visible cause, even in the case of mediums who can produce them at will. All these peculiarities make it difficult to persuade the mediums to conform to the exact methods of experimental psychology, the more so as they are very sensitive people who are quite aware if they are being approached in a spirit of distrust ; and feel at once whether the experimenters are going to " show up the fraud " or whether they are kindly disposed towards them. This is not at all the same thing as being uncritical. One would expect psychologists to know that there is no similar feat of intellect which does not require its own particular conditions ; this comprehension of the required conditions is generally lacking in dealing with mediums. They must be treated as very sensitive and unstable beings if good results are to be attained, just as the standard of work done by school children varies enormously with the way in which they are approached. Ordinary intellectual work such as arithmetic, etc., may not be much affected by moods, environment, and other similar factors, but it is doubtful whether Goethe would have been able to allay suspicions as to his capacity for writing verse by making beautiful poems in a psychological laboratory. Subconscious work of this type cannot be produced at will ; nor can these mediumistic faculties, which are closely bound up with the subconscious, take place to order, for their emergence out of the subconscious seems to depend on the chance of the moment.

Owing to the way in which a great many of them have been treated, mediumistic circles tend to fight shy of the scientific investigation of their powers. Some, of course, do so for very different reasons. You cannot simply ask a medium to come to a psychological laboratory on such and such a day at this or that time to be put to the test ; you have to get to know him gradually, to gain his confidence by degrees ; you can only think of improving or altering the conditions of the experiments when this has been attained, and this must then be done very slowly, in the hope of obtaining results under test conditions. I had the good fortune to come in touch with, and to experiment upon, several persons possessing this faculty. Except in the first instance, it was only after years of patient research that I was able to find suitable mediums. I had plenty of opportunity of sorting the chaff from the grain, of trying to eliminate fraud and illusion. It sounds very well, and gives the impression of real scientific judgment, when a scientist states from his armchair that he could surely have found out the trick. Much weight is given to experience in science ; it might be as well here, too, to credit the experienced worker with a little judgment on the subject, and not to think, as is often the case, that the investigator in occult matters is possessed of less intelligence and a weaker critical faculty than the average man. The question of morality should also be accepted without preconceived ideas. It is not fair to behave like the judge who considered that any prisoner in the dock who pleaded not guilty of the crime he was accused of, was particularly open to suspicion ; nor should we regard every investigator who has satisfied himself that a series of occult phenomena is genuine as open to suspicion as a " mystic ", and condemn him accordingly.

Who is the expert in this field ? The philosopher ? the psychologist ? the neurologist ? or the conjurer ? I deny to every one of them singly, and all of them together, the right to call themselves experts in psychical research. But to be able to pronounce a judgment in occult matters you must have a certain amount of the knowledge of the philosopher, the psychologist, the neurologist, and the conjurer. Nor is that all ; you must have a good practical experience of the subject in general, and of mediums in particular, as well as a thorough knowledge of the literature. Only then can you hope to be able to apply unbiassed scientific thought to the problems in hand. If anyone sits down in his study and plans a series of experiments which he hopes to carry out as such to the last detail, and without any concessions to the medium, he will probably fail. Often you have to slacken the reins, but without losing hold of them. It is quite useless to try to enforce your will on the medium from the very beginning. Tamers no longer tame animals with the whip, but investigators of the occult often think it necessary to tame mediums by using force. I think I can show that it is possible to obtain satisfactory results by conceding a point occasionally, by taking into account the whims of the medium in the choice of methods. Nor are their scarcity, their unreliability, and the possibilities of fraud which they present the *only* reasons that make psychic phenomena have such a hard fight for acceptance. There are other causes as well. Psychic phenomena do not yet fit into the edifice of natural science ; they cannot be derived from its laws and hypothesis; they form, as it were, a foreign body in its organism. This is why there is a tendency to deny the existence of the facts themselves because we cannot explain them. Whenever there is a possibility of explaining the facts we find people ready to accept them as possible or as true. Ostwald, for instance, thinks that he can explain certain facts of occultism by means of his energetics. Forel states in a recent publication (*Journal für Psychologie und Neurologie*, 1918) that the facts of wireless telegraphy have for some time enabled him to accept by analogy the possibility of telepathy.

It is already a step in the right direction, when a

scientist is prepared to recognize this subject, but it would be a much greater advance if his hypotheses were found to be correct and to provide the necessary explanations. It is easy to understand that the inexplicable should be rejected, but that does not make the rejection any more permissible. Must it be the empiricist, so proud of differing from the philosopher who recognizes the a priori, who should refute a real a priori judgment in this case, a judgment in which the assumption that he already knows all the laws of nature is dogmatically contained ? How does he know that all his knowledge is final, that he will not one day have to pull down large parts of the edifice of science and build them up afresh ? The laws of nature have not been impressed on it from the outside ; they have been deduced, or, as it were, extracted from the phenomena of nature, and have had to be altered many a time to fit them.

But the cause of the aversion is a deeper one. Not only do the laws of nature seem to be shaken by these facts, but fundamental principles on which both philosophy and science are based are apparently in danger. *Nihil est in intellectu quod non antea fuerit in sensibus* is one of the fundamental principles of critical philosophy ; it says that the whole content of our minds is derived from data which are based on perceptions which we have received through our senses. Important systems of philosophy go so far as to state that not only the content but the form of thought, i.e. its laws and categories, are all derived from sensual experience. In fact, both the main directions of thought agree that the content of our thought is based on experience gained in that way.

The whole of modern epistemology and metaphysics, and by far the greater part of modern philosophy, are based on this principle. Science itself is built up on facts gained through the senses and has gradually led us to consider that all we can accept as scientifically true is derived from sense-perceptions and never from pure thought. Can we be surprised if science tries to reject a study which seems to involve the destruction of the whole edifice ? From this point of view we can even understand how the American biologist mentioned above could say that no effort should be spared to destroy and hide the facts of telepathy, though we may condemn his point of view. William James himself, and on this I would lay particular stress, was quite convinced of the reality of these phenomena, thanks to his own experiences, and has many a hard word for his colleagues who closed their eyes to these facts and could not find time to study them (*Proc. S.P.R.*, 1901–2, xvii, 13–23).

It is obvious that once telepathy and clairvoyance are accepted, the reign of sense-experience is at an end. The moment we can refer facts to another criterion than that of the outer senses, sense-experience will have to come down from her throne.

But will it really shake philosophy and science to their very foundations ? I do not think that this apparent destruction would be final, for a slight change in the fundamental principles would probably avert the danger. Even if telepathy and clairvoyance cannot be regarded as sensuous-experience, they can be regarded as a form of experience. If we discriminate between sensuous and extra-sensuous or super-sensuous experience, the main principles will be saved. It may in some cases complicate the methods of scientific investigation, but these faculties are rare, and in most cases they will not come into the question at all. However, scientists cannot afford to neglect this study, just as they cannot afford to neglect disturbing factors in their experiments simply because they are inconvenient to deal with.

Not only will the path of experience be a different

one, but its content will also change in many respects. Not only will a number of strange facts confront us, but perhaps new forms of energy and natural factors hitherto unknown ; as has often happened in science. We may recall the Röntgen Rays, which were most startling and not quite easy to fit into existing theories, and Radium, which seemed to undermine that fundamental law of natural science " the conservation of energy ", but which was finally fitted into the edifice of science.

The attraction of a piece of iron by a magnet, if regarded as an isolated fact, is a contradiction of the law of gravity, but if we presuppose a new kind of energy we can explain it easily. We shall probably come across the same principle in occult problems. We must bear this in mind, and not be too ready to say that an exception to the laws of nature is unthinkable ; the opinion held by so many sceptics that the facts of occultism are in opposition to the laws of nature should not disconcert us, as we shall probably find when we go deeper into these questions that other forms of energy, governed by other laws, come into action and modify or eliminate the action of the laws we are familiar with ; just as the action of the law of gravity is cancelled by the action of magnetism. All such a priori objections as have been made lately by Robert Meyer [1] are beside the point : it is not permissible to use the law of causality as an argument against the possibility of clairvoyance into the future (second-sight), by saying that cause and effect cannot change

---

[1] In the *Berliner Klinische Wochenschrift*, " It is," he says, "'impossible' and ' unthinkable ' for us to assume that an exception or a contradiction to the laws of nature could exist. We cannot afford to drop this principle, and the man who does not accept it is guilty of being illogical, or of believing in a superstition, or both." Meyer presupposes that we know all the laws of nature, whereas what we call the laws of nature are surely but fragmentary and often erroneous interpretations; as it were, " readings " of true events.

places. Anyone who is inclined to agree with Robert Meyer in regarding the law of causality as existing a priori, as a postulate, would agree with him that a contradiction of that law is an impossibility ; but would certainly contend that this does not force us to admit the alternative—either contradiction of the law of causality or agreement with it. If the law is considered in this way the decision would be an easy one, and would be against the existence of the phenomena of occultism. It seems to me most unlikely that the existence of second-sight should be regarded as a blow to the law of causality ; it involves no inversion of cause and effect. I cannot see that the facts point to that conclusion, much less force it upon us. If we accept second-sight as a fact, and look at it empirically, we find it to be a foreknowledge of events, due to impressions received, which are probably of a super-normal nature. It is comparable to the case of a doctor telling a patient that he will suffer from loco-motor-ataxy in a few years on the strength of a few symptoms. The patient not being aware of the symptoms finds the doctor's prediction quite unin-telligible. No one will dream of considering this a reversal of cause and effect. The case of second-sight is probably similar, though more difficult to under-stand, as we do not know the intermediate links. This does not, however, justify Meyer's rejection of second-sight as nonsense. It is a question of empirical facts and cannot be disproved by a simple negation on a priori grounds. This is a typical example of the point of view adopted by many towards occultism.

It would serve no practical purpose to seek further for true explanations in this domain, since too little is known about the facts. It will suffice for the present to remind the reader that it has always been possible to fit new facts into the body of science in such a way that they really became a part of it. Even if some of the fundamental principles have to be modified, it will not cause the newly-gained experience to lose its value if rightly understood, or the laws of science to be destroyed.

Hypnotism is a parallel case. The facts were not accepted for a long time, and had a pitiful existence outside the realm of science under the name of " mesmerism " or " animal magnetism ". But hypnotism—the occultism of yesterday—has at last found its place among the sciences, and is not open to doubt any longer. I would not, however, go so far as to say that is has found its true place, or that it is looked upon in its true light.

Let us try to imagine what would be the importance and function of telepathy and clairvoyance in everyday life, if these faculties were common. The idea of the inventor would not be safe in his head, the plan of action of the general would be known to his opponents at once, the contents of every safe could be seen, man would no longer be alone in his thoughts and actions. I will not depict any further consequences ; they would be far-reaching indeed, both to the advantage and the disadvantage of the individual and of the community. We should adapt ourselves gradually to these new facts, and in the long run the good results would surpass the evil ones. However, we need not fear any great change; these faculties are much too rare and much too partial. It matters little whether a phenomenon is rare in science, but whether it is true or not. If this is the case we must accept the phenomenon as a fact, and draw the necessary practical and theoretical consequences, which may be similar to those we draw in practical life, but which will surely not render the continuance of science impossible.

On the one hand, then, we have Science treating this whole study most critically, even with a strong bias against it ; on the other a by no means negligible stream of thought, namely, Theosophy no longer regarding these facts as a problem or as requiring inductive proof. From the standpoint of the latter, they are the natural outcome of certain views according to which they not only *can* but *must* exist ; it is quite useless to give up one's time to these problems, or to collect scientific material ; nor is it desirable, for it would be a waste of time ; and it is considered a violation of personality to put a medium into trance for purposes of study.

Occultism is, as it were, squeezed in between these two currents of thought, and does not get enough air to expand and bear fruit. But the very friends of occultism are often its greatest enemies, more terrible than the two classes just mentioned ; for by far the greater number of occultists bring the subject into discredit owing to a lack of critical faculty.

It will be obvious by now that it is my aim to interpret occultism in a purely scientific and non-mystical manner. I will consider, therefore, the relation of critical occultism to the non-critical, mystical occultism. To my mind, occultism is a field of knowledge like any other ; it has its peculiarities, and they must be taken into account. It is certainly rich in vague conceptions and is interwoven essentially with mysticism, but this mysticism is not an intrinsic part of it. Occultism, as I understand it, is closely related to ecstasy, to mystical meditation and allied phenomena, but we must draw the line between the investigation of these facts from a scientific point of view and their use in the interests of any philosophical or religious views. This should in no case be attempted, except as the last link of a chain, and knowing that it is an *interpretation* of these facts which is being attempted. In my opinion, these facts still need much study and thought; they can be interpreted in different ways, so that we shall do well to be very wary in converting them into philosophical or religious thought. Quite apart from that, it seems to me that we are confusing two different realms when we try to prove scientifically our religious beliefs. A religion which requires a scientific proof seems to me to be lacking in persuasive power.

B. The Position of the Problem

I should like, at the outset, to indicate the state of the subject when I started my work, and at the same time to give a short survey of some of the later Continental work, and the way in which it has been criticized. My work is purely experimental, but it may be useful to mention a few publications which are not of a strictly experimental nature.

Dr. Bock, of Munich, published in 1913, in the *Süddeutsche Monatshefte*, a number of instances in which he had supernormal knowledge of coming events. Some of the cases seem to be due to telepathic influences, some to a clairvoyance in space and time similar to second-sight. In most cases the visions are so detailed that chance is quite out of the question ; for instance, he saw a relative of his, who was about to undergo an operation, lying in a particular room in hospital, which he recognized quite distinctly. He knew that another room had been ordered for her, and rang up the hospital to make sure that she should be given the room ordered. He had seen her wearing a coloured ribbon. His relative was operated on ; the room she was to have had was not ready, as the patient still in it could not be removed, and when he came to see her she was lying in the room as he had seen her, and wearing the coloured ribbon. He says that he can rely on the accuracy of his visions. For instance, he saw his mother dying ; her death was quite unexpected, but he packed up his things and made all preparations for the journey, although he had not yet received telegraphic notice of the fact.

The Viennese clairvoyant, Raphael Schermann, is generally inspired by writing, but the statements he makes are often connected with the past or future life of the writer, and do not bear a graphological character. The first experimental work we shall consider is that of the Russian doctor, Naum Kotik. It was published in 1908 under the title *Die Emanation der psychophysischen Energie* (Munich). He made a number of experiments in both telepathy and clairvoyance. Kotik was the agent. A girl of fourteen, known as Lydia, the percipient, was in the same room and gave her answers by automatic writing.

Here are a few examples ; the first word is the word transmitted, the second is the answer given :

Loschadj (horse)	Loschadj
Pole (field)	Trawa (grass)
Nikolaus (proper name)	Nikolaus
Swonok (bell)	Swonok
Gaseta (newspaper)	Journal.

Lydia does not always give the right word, but probably has an intuitive perception of the object (journal) or of something closely associated with it (trawa).

Kotik also tried experiments in clairvoyance, and in these too the medium gave her answers in automatic writing. He asked friends to give him letters containing short sentences describing some definite thought expressed concisely, e.g. :

" A crowd walks down the street carrying a red flag."

Answer. " A dull sound . . . like a murmuring crowd . . . something gigantic comes rolling along . . . an unusual scene . . . there is something quiet and majestic in this procession of the people."

17

Finally Kotik tried some experiments with " thought laden paper ". He asked some friends to hold a blank sheet of paper in their hands, and to look intently at a picture postcard at the same time. The blank sheet was put into an envelope and sent to Kotik, the friend keeping the postcard for comparison. Here is the report of one of these experiments :

Object. A blank sheet of paper (in an envelope or just taken out of it by the medium). The original postcard represented a broad band of coastline in the foreground ; fields, woods, in the centre a monastery with many cupolas, and the sea in the background.

Answer. " Bright green fields . . . a wood seems to be coming out green in the distance . . . between the trees a number of buildings . . . several cupolas are visible . . . then a smooth sheet of water . . . it seems to be the sea."

Sceptics have found fault with Kotik's work in many ways, and there may be points in which it is open to criticism ; but a great many of the experiments seem to me beyond criticism. Chance, tricks, and other kinds of fraud cannot provide adequate explanations of the results of these experiments, although they might have been more fully reported.

Professor Schottelius published a report of experiments he had made with a clairvoyant in the *Journal für Psychologie und Neurologie* (vol. xx) in 1913, which caused a great sensation. This clairvoyant, a Mr. Kahn, aged 40, of Jewish origin, was able to read folded slips, which the investigator had written in his absence and held in his closed hand all the time, or had in his pocket, or under a blotting-pad on the table. Meyer, in his criticism of these experiments (*Berliner Klinische Wochenschrift*, 1914, No. 32), tries to make it seem likely that Kahn was able to see the contents of the slips either by exchanging them or by distracting the attention of the investigator. Several different experimenters, however, emphatically affirmed that Kahn never had the slips in his hand ; they were written when he was not in the room and either held in the hand of the investigator or put in a book or other place where he could not see them. Meyer himself never made one single experiment with Kahn, and it is not at all clear on what facts he bases his criticism.[1] In 1913 Dr. W. von Wasielewski published in the *Annalen für Natur u. Kulturphilosophie*, a series of experiments performed with a Miss von B. I have also had the pleasure of doing some experiments with Miss v. B., which are published in this book. She had the gift of describing, and often of drawing, objects carefully packed ; this she often did under conditions which made fraud impossible. Dr. v. Wasielewski almost always knew the object, and telepathy cannot be considered excluded in most cases ; but the experiments, which were very carefully planned and carried out, certainly prove the existence of supernormal faculties. The results seem to be due to clairvoyance in the majority of the cases.

This was the state of things when I wrote my book. Various publications have appeared since, which I should like to mention briefly. Baron von Schrenck-Notzing published a German translation (Munich, 1919) of Dr. Chowrin's book on clairvoyance just before the publication of my book. The original Russian edition had appeared in 1898, but had attracted hardly any attention, and it was the translation which really brought the book before the eye of the public. Chowrin describes experiments done with a lady who could read the contents of closed letters. The most interesting

[1] Similar statements have been made by persons concerning phenomena which without any doubt were fraudulent. In this connexion the classical experiments of Dr. Richard Hodgson with Mr. Davey may be consulted. (*Proc. S.P.R.*, 1886–7, pt. xi.) [*Trans.*]

characteristic of her clairvoyance from a psychological point of view was that she did not read the writing, but saw the scenes described, as visions. The experiments were very carefully conducted, some of them taking place in the presence of the experimenter himself, and the results obtained cannot be explained by chance, guesswork, or fraud. It is a pity that Dr. Chowrin's theoretical point of view was so limited ; he tried to explain all his results by hyperæsthesia of the senses, whereas it is obvious that most of them cannot possibly be explained in this way. He was so sure that his theory was right that he never tried to exclude the possibility of hyperæsthesia.

In 1921 Dr. von Wasielewski published a book, *Telepathie und Hellsehen* (Halle), in which he describes all his previous experiments and a number of new ones with Miss v. B. All kinds of different experiments on clairvoyance are included : telæsthesia, cryptoscopy, microscopical clairvoyance, psychometry, as well as further experiments on telepathy.

Another book on clairvoyance, called *Seelisches Erfühlen* (Pfullingen), by Dr. Böhm, contains a series of experiments with one medium. It is most unfortunate that the author does not report all his experiments, as it would have been interesting to calculate the proportion of successful ones. The results seem to be due to a mixture of telepathy and clairvoyance ; this is shown by the fact that the answers often do not correspond to the object under consideration, but refer to ideas that one or other of the sitters, often Böhm himself, had about the object. The medium often expressed himself by mimicry, either copying the movements of the owners of the object or movements connected with the object itself ; for instance, he imitated the movements of a monkey when holding a parcel containing a monkey's paw.

Finally, I would mention Dr. Geley's experiments with a Polish engineer Ossowiecki (*Revue, Métapsychique*, 1921, Nos. 5 and 8), who showed a strong clairvoyant, and especially psychometric, faculty. Ossowiecki does not see the drawing that is given him wrapped up, but receives an impression of the object itself, which he then proceeds to draw ; in one case he drew a fish quite different from the original drawing (the original was long with a great many scales, Ossowiecki's short and fat with few scales).

I will now give a short survey of the utterances of some of the best known scientists and critics of occultism ; a survey which makes no claim to be exhaustive.

Wundt mentions telepathy and clairvoyance casually in his three volume *Physiologische Psychologie*. He speaks of "this so-called telepathy" and "similar aberrations". Jodl, the philosopher, speaks of the fabulous and sentimental idea that there should be such a thing as telepathy in his *Lehrbuch der Psychologie* (vol. ii, p. 23). And again : " Such a direct transmission of ideas from one mind to another, without any perceptible physical method of communication, would indicate the presence of a crack in the very foundations of all our views on nature, and if because the proofs were so conclusive we had to recognize its existence it would lead us to a complete revision of fundamental principles " (vol. ii, p. 165). H. Henning, in the *Journal für Psychologie u. Neurologie*, vol. xxiii, says : "Psycho-physics, yes, even psychology, as a science must be utterly wrecked before we have recourse to telepathy." It is not at all obvious why telepathy should be placed in such exclusive opposition to science. Kohnstamm says telepathy is "impossible". Among neurologists we have Löwenfeld, who is inclined to accept it, not to mention Forel, to whom we have previously referred.

The two authors who have gone more deeply into

the subject, Max Dessoir (*Vom Jenseits der Seele*, Stuttgart, 1917) and R. Hennig (*Wunder der Wissenschaft*, Hamburg, 1904), seem more favourably inclined. But the impression remains that they do not judge it quite justly. They seem to emphasize the negative evidence, and to judge the positive results too severely ; neither of them considers telepathy or clairvoyance as proved. To me Dessoir's criticism of Kotik's work seems biassed and not justified by the facts ; he caricatures the experiments, for he does not mention that the answers in the experiments he alludes to are quite characteristic of the objects ; neither does he describe the latter. He also neglects to state that the fact of the description of the first example and the answer to the fourth, which he quotes, fitting each other is due to the two postcards in these particular experiments being very similar (p. 118). The reader must get a very false and inadequate impression of the value of Kotik's experiments from the fact that Professor Dessoir only mentions a few of them. I would not claim that Kotik's experiments were perfect, but he did not deserve to be treated so cavalierly.

M. Hopp (*Ueber Hellsehen*, Dissertation, Königsberg, 1916) wrote an essay on clairvoyance in which he sharply criticized the attempts to prove the existence of clairvoyance up to his time. He then goes on to say that there is no reason why science should go to the trouble of investigating the matter at first hand ; it is quite enough for it to criticize the evidence as it is published. It would seem that he considers the probability of clairvoyance really existing as very slight, otherwise his point of view would be almost incomprehensible, given the importance of the subject (see above, Jodl and Henning).

I am not aware that any of the better-known modern textbooks on psychology accepts these facts or even considers them at any length. Earlier, things were different. For instance J. H. Fichte's *Anthropologie* (3rd edition, 1876), and his *Psychologie* (1864), devote about ten per cent of each book to the subject and accept it as real. Now, we are in a strange vicious circle. The subject is neglected because it is supposed not to exist, and this neglect prevents its existence being proved. I do not think that ten per cent of the philosophers in Germany know the meaning of psychometry, control, exteriorization of sensibility, or have heard of Myers and Mrs. Piper.

It is only quite lately that a change has begun to take place. Telepathy and clairvoyance are beginning to be accepted by a few. I would particularly mention three philosophers in this connexion : Professor Hans Driesch, who has tried to draw the attention of the public to this subject in his *Wirklichkeitslehre* (Leipzig, 1917), and *Die Westmark* (1921, 7) ; Professor T. K. Oesterreich, *Der Okkultismus im Modernen Weltbild* (Dresden, 1921), and finally Graf Hermann Keyserling, *Reisetagebuch eines Philosophen* (Munich, 1919).

It has been said that science can only accept as facts such phenomena as may be reproduced at will by any experimenter at any time, and in any place. Of course, it does lead us to a more intimate knowledge of the facts to be able to study phenomena that can be produced and varied at will. This is very rarely the case in occultism, but rather can artistic inspiration or ecstasy be produced to order in a laboratory. In some of the sciences also, meteorology and astronomy for instance, we are dependent on chance for the study of certain phenomena ; and yet nobody, for that reason, dreams of contesting their right to a place among the sciences.

Certain medical phenomena have been observed but rarely, or only once, and yet they have been incorporated in the body of medicine ; such observations are usually regarded as accurate if the observer is known to have done reliable work. This degree of faith in observations would not be necessary in many observations of the supernormal. Whole series of experiments have been made with more than one medium, and the results obtained were similar, and consistent with one another. So there seems no adequate reason for putting these facts outside the realm of science ; a great many occult phenomena can be reproduced within certain limits. Of course the authority of the experimenters in occultism, and the faith reposed in them, will have to be great. At the beginning it can be lessened, but not dispensed with. To obviate this objection, I have tried my best from the beginning to induce other scientists to be present at the experiments. Becher von Aster, Baensch, and Gallinger, professors of philosophy, and Specht and Gruber, professors of medicine, all witnessed successful experiments. In the last year's work reported in this book most of the experiments took place in the presence of a medical Commission, called into existence after a lecture I gave before the Medical Society. I cannot present an official certificate proving the scientific integrity of each of the members of this commission, but those of my readers who do not know by reputation the scientists mentioned will have to be satisfied with the fact that such a medical society would not appoint scientists of doubtful capacity to check my experiments ; and this fact should bring with it some degree of guarantee that the arrangement of my experiments was satisfactory, and that the results can be relied on. If the experiments done in the presence of the medical commission and approved by them can be relied on, then we may take it that the experiments carried out in their absence with similar results are reliable also. So we have our premises that the observed phenomena are accurate, and we must proceed to test whether the logical discussion of this raw material is satisfactory.

INTRODUCTORY

I cannot give as long a series of experiments as is usual in the other sciences, but I hope the number will be sufficient to carry this science a little further, especially considering the difficult conditions which prevail in occultism.

I would particularly draw attention to the fact that I have published the results of all my experiments on telepathy and clairvoyance with the three mediums, Miss von B., Mr. R., and Mr. H., in this book, and so these series must not in any case be considered as specially chosen. The reader can see for himself that the percentage of successful experiments is really fairly high.

These experiments were made under differing conditions, and they vary in value ; if anyone wishes to consider them critically, he should attach most weight to those carried out under the strictest conditions, not on the poorer ones. If the former prove the existence of genuine supernormal phenomena, then he can consider the results of the experiments done under less stringent conditions, but with similar results, as showing phenomena of the same class. Only a partial critic would neglect the above considerations, laying stress only on the lack of neatness of some of the experiments, or on my attempts to class them as positive or negative, expecially those on psychoscopy, and would omit to mention the really successful ones. Facts are of primary importance at this stage, and I fully realize that theory is a secondary matter. Nevertheless I have given up considerable space to it. But I hope that anyone who does not share my theories will remember that they can never alter the facts.

II

EXPERIMENTS

A. Telepathy

I TOOK no active interest in supernormal phenomena until 1912. My acquaintance with the subject was limited to the reading of a few books and essays, and to the witnessing of a few table-turning sittings. My attitude was not one of a priori opposition or negation, but rather of cautious expectation. This line of thought was really opened up to me through meeting Professor L. Staudenmaier, author of *Die Magie als Experimentelle Naturwissenschaft* (Leipzig, 1912), who also lived in Freising. At about the same time, i.e. in the latter half of 1912, I received a letter from my friend Dr. W. von Wasielewski, telling me of some experiments on telepathy he had made with Miss v. B., a lady of his acquaintance. In October, 1912, he came to stay with me in Freising, and told me more about his experiments, which interested me greatly. We decided then and there to ask Miss v. B. to come to Freising for some further experiments. She kindly accepted our invitation.

As we had not mentioned to one another our intentions of publishing our results, we both felt at liberty to include them in a treatise on the subject. When we realized that both of us had done so, we decided to leave things as they were ; in fact, it seemed rather a good thing that two independent descriptions of experiments should have been published, using the same records as a foundation.

EXPERIMENTS

Our first series of experiments dealt mainly with telepathy, as we had no idea that Miss v. B. was gifted with clairvoyance. I conducted the séance, chose the objects, and kept the records, but in order to save time, refrained from acting as agent.

The experiments were carried out as follows : we put a three-panelled screen covered with a thick rug round three sides of my writing-table chair. The rug acted as a roof and hung down the sides, so that it would have been quite impossible to see anything through the chinks in the screen. The table at which Dr. v. Wasielewski and I sat was from ten to twelve feet behind the back of this chair. Miss v. B. sat down in this chair while the doctor and I adjourned to a distant room on the same landing. We subsequently went upstairs to a bedroom where we chose the objects, pausing in several other rooms on our return so as to make it impossible for the medium to know in which room we had chosen the objects for the experiments. Before letting the doctor come in with the object chosen for a particular experiment, I made sure that Miss v. B. was seated in her chair. The doctor sat down back to back with her, and about nine feet away. I sat facing him in such a position that I could see the screen behind him, and could notice any attempt on the part of the medium to look round the screen. I never once saw her do so during the frequent intervals when I was not writing. Even if she had tried to see the object she would have failed, as it was hidden from her by the doctor's body. I got up several times and crept to a place whence I could see what she was doing, and every time I looked she was sitting quietly with her legs crossed. We did not hypnotize Miss v. B., nor did she go into a trance, but maintained full consciousness throughout the experiments. I must add that there were no mirrors or bright surfaces in the room.

TELEPATHY AND CLAIRVOYANCE

We meant to begin our experiments after dinner, but made a few trials before, which I will mention for the sake of completeness.

1st Experiment. Time 6–7 p.m. Object : a shaving-brush. " Dark—longish, round—as if from a bouquet—as if from a branch—a curious thing—like a small stick. Like leather." (Dr. v. W. : " How do you mean like leather ? ") " As if made of leather—cannot be a fruit—it is very difficult to tell—now it is getting coloured—vividly coloured." *Negative.*

2nd Experiment. Object: a pair of scissors. Miss v.B. had just stated that it was made of metal, when we were called in to dinner. We locked up the scissors[1] and did not allude to the experiment during dinner. After dinner, when Miss v. B. had settled down on her chair behind the screen, we took the scissors out of the drawer and continued the experiment. Miss v. B. did not know we were going on with the experiment.

8.14$\frac{3}{4}$ p.m. Dr. v. W. takes up the scissors.

8.16$\frac{3}{4}$. Miss v. B. says : " Seems to be very large—I am still very much taken up with my thoughts—now it seems to be a small narrow thing—it is very difficult to identify."

8.21$\frac{1}{2}$. " I am afraid I am very absent-minded—to-day's impressions keep cropping up—now I see one of Mrs. Tischner's pictures—is it a coin ? " (Dr. v. W. : " No.")

8.22$\frac{1}{2}$. " It is getting round and shiny—keeps on shining—now it is becoming like a ring."

8.24. " It is still made of metal—shines like metal or glass—round and yet long—as if it were a pair of scissors—there are two round things at the bottom, and then it gets long."

---

[1] The scissors were locked up in the roll-top writing desk in my study; we adjourned to the dining-room at once and did not return to my study till we continued the experiment.

8.26½. "Must be a pair of scissors—(then with certainty) it is a pair of scissors." *Positive.*

3rd Experiment. Object : a violin. The doctor is a good violinist, so you will believe me when I say that he did not touch the strings by mistake and simplify the "telepathy".

8.36½ p.m. The experiment begins.

8.37¾. "It seems to be small—longish—rounded—dull-coloured."

8.39. "Reddish—yellowish—reminds one of an egg—like an elongated sphere—oval—dull reddish yellow, like a ball : but it isn't a ball."

8.42½. "Like a dyed egg, but it has a dark spot on the top of it."

8.43¼. "Now it looks like a fruit, probably a pear, now it is lengthening considerably."

8.45½. "It is bright red now"—(Dr. v. W. : "Is it not getting clearer or larger?")—"It is getting quite dark—something long with a handle with a twist at the end—getting large—what can it be ?—It has got still larger and has light streaks on it. It looks as if made of dark wood—rounded at the bottom, and has a long handle which is twisted at the end like a snail's shell.—Now it looks as if it were a violin."

8.49. "It must be a violin—looks like a violin"—(Dr. v. W. : "What colour?")—"brown"—(Now the doctor says : "We will only proceed with this experiment for a short time, so as not to tire you, and then stop," so as to try and mislead her).—(In rather an offended tone) "I can't help it, it really does look like a violin." *Positive.*

4th Experiment. Object : a conical flask of greenish flashed glass with a conical stopper.

The flask was not taken into the room. Dr. v. W. looked at it carefully in the dining-room ; we went to the bedroom, stayed there for some time, and came back to my study. Miss v. B. was sitting at the table, with the doctor about five feet from her at right angles and opposite to me.

9.16½ p.m.

9.19. " How plastic it looks ! "

9.21. " Looks like a figure, and yet it does not—I think it will be very difficult this time."

9.23. " Not like a picture—more like something plastic."

9.24. " The whole thing is very bright, and there is something in the middle which looks like glass or silvered plate glass, like a building or a figure. Like a figure with an appendage. It is curiously long—with a figure to the right and one to the left. It glistens every now and again—there must be some water connected with it—a form is placed on something—it rises gradually "—(T. : " In what way ")—" it is low on the sides and rises gradually."

9.29. " It still looks as if there were water, more so in the middle than outside—there is a figure on each side—looks as if it was made of some light stone—I keep on seeing water or something bright."

9.31½. The doctor moves up to her side and takes hold of her left hand, as the experiment is not progressing satisfactorily.

9.32. " I can't help it—I still see it glistening—now I see a form—something riding on an animal."

9.35. A pause.

9.37. " A bowl of water—a big bowl—more water—three forms—forms riding and water."

The doctor and I went to fetch the object. He went quite gently into the room next but one and fetched the flask out of the cupboard, while I tramped upstairs. We did this to obviate any possibility of Miss v. B. getting any clues. I made sure that she was sitting in her niche so that she could see neither door nor table ; then the doctor came in, keeping the object hidden till we were both seated as in the previous experiments.

9.39. (Almost immediately) " I see it more clearly —it glistens—it shines like water."

9.41. " It is something tall which sparkles in the middle—I don't see any more figures."

We had not told the medium whether she was right or wrong ; we had only said that the experiment would get on better if we fetched the object.

" The object is taller than it is broad—it sparkles tremendously—seems polished—it is taking shape— like a ninepin—like a bottle, but it sparkles tremendously. It glistens like water, and yet it is coloured —as if it were green—like a green bottle glistening in the middle. It must be polished."

9.45. " A cut-glass flask—but much narrower than it is broad. A tall thin flask—green and white—made of glass."

The description of the object given after it had been fetched was very good. " It glistens like water and yet it is coloured " describes flashed glass perfectly. *Positive.*

5th Experiment. Object : a drawing.

I just want to mention a single experiment, the only successful one on telepathy done with a Miss S., from Munich. We had chosen a number of figures between one and nine, and she had given some of them correctly, but not more than we should be led to expect according to the theory of probabilities ; so I omit the record here.

Before I made her acquaintance, Miss S. had attended a few table-turning séances, at which she had fallen into trance. We had two sittings together, and I will publish an experiment tried in the first one later on, when we reach the category to which it belongs.

The second sitting was a very long table-turning séance, at which a French soldier, who was still alive— an acquaintance of Miss S.'s—said that he was in control. At last Miss S. fell into trance. As the table-turning did not interest me, I broke it off and gave a small drawing to a friend of hers, with whom she had declared herself to be in telepathic communication several times. This lady was seated facing Miss S., at a distance of about 9 feet, with the drawing in front of her, protected from Miss S.'s view by a book. The medium was in deep trance. Her eyes were tightly shut, and I was able to ascertain that her eyeballs were turned up, so we took no further precautions, as it was quite impossible for her to see the drawing.

"Two rectangles—a small one like the sign of the Jews—a rectangle, a small one—a triangle."

I asked her to draw what she saw : I put a pencil in her hand, which was quite limp, and then held a piece of paper on her lap, the paper lying on the flat of my hand. I think that this sketch, drawn with closed eyes, is a surprisingly positive test, which could not possibly be referred to chance. *Positive*.

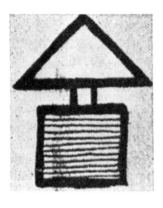

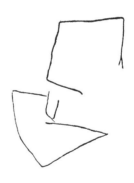

FIG. 1.   FIG. 2.

At our later sittings I put her into trance with a few passes, as she took such a long time to fall into trance, but got no decisive results.

EXPERIMENTS

Discussion of the Results

As we have seen, all the experiments except No. 1 were solved without a single mistake. The main question is : Has fraud played any part in it all ? Have any points been neglected which should have influenced a clear judgment on this series of experiments ? Are there any illusions or mistakes which play an important part without our being aware of them ? Can one or several of these factors explain all our results, or are we obliged to conclude that the information was gained by telepathy or at any rate by some super-sensuous means ? The first question is whether the persons taking part in the experiments were reliable. It is generally taken for granted that the experimenters, in this case Wasielewski and I, are trustworthy men, trying their best to obtain reliable data, unless any facts proving the contrary have been brought up against us. Readers with whom we are not personally acquainted can only form an opinion on the subject for themselves by reading our books and other publications. Of course this can never exclude the possibility of objective lack of veracity, i.e. error or deception.

Naturally, I can offer no absolute proof of the trustworthiness and reliability of Miss von B. But I fancy that the arrangement of the experiments made it almost impossible for Miss von B. to obtain sensuous knowledge of the objects even had she wanted to, and so did away with a great many possible sources of error. But there are other factors which speak strongly against any cause for distrust. The medium was never hypnotized and never fell into trance, which puts unconscious fraud, as it is known in such cases, out of the question. She gave the impression of having sound nerves and a sound mind, without any signs of hysteria. This impression was corroborated by what

33

TELEPATHY AND CLAIRVOYANCE

I heard about her from her relatives, and by what I saw of her later on when she stayed at our house and I at hers. Hysteria would surely have shown itself somewhere. So I think I can safely say that she was not hysterical, and had no tendency to lying or deception. She showed no signs of trying to make herself interesting by reason of so unusual a faculty, as many hysterical people do. This tendency and the desire for fame were entirely absent ; she was rather shy of showing her faculties and always had to be persuaded to try experiments ; whereas she was full of life and keenly interested in other matters, so that this lack of interest in her special faculty was somewhat contradictory. Finally we have to consider the pecuniary interest she may have had in the experiments, and it must, therefore, be admitted that she had some coffee and cake, a dinner, and a glass of wine at my house.

The theory of telepathy itself will be considered later ; here I would only deal with what Lehmann and Hansen called the " whispering theory of telepathy ", which to me is not a theory but mainly a source of error. They stated in their paper in *Philosophische Studien*, vol. ii, that a semblance of telepathy could be given by involuntary and unconscious whispering. This so-called theory has been used so often to throw discredit on this whole study that I think it might be well to consider it in detail, especially as Lehmann and Hansen thought they found the corroboration of their theory in one of Sidgwick's publications, in which they tried to show that the mistakes made in the transmission of messages were due to words being wrongly heard. They made a series of experiments which in the mouth of the agent and the ear of the percipient were in the foci of parallel concave mirrors ; they say that they once tried " not to check the involuntary tendency to whisper ". Certainly this comes very near to actual involuntary whispering, and then again to actual whispering, and it can easily happen that an a priori theory may seem thus to be proved.

Hansen and Lehmann were so sure of the correctness of their theory that Lehmann went so far as to write in his book *Aberglaube u. Zauberei* (1st edition, p. 461) the sentence : " Now we know that thought transference depends on unconscious whispering." I am sure that any occultist who got to " know " anything so quickly would be condemned at once. Hansen goes on to say, for instance, that it was due to a mistake of auditive perception that 7 and 0 were mistaken for one another in Sidgwick's experiments. He calls them seven and zero. Sidgwick drew his attention to the fact that " 0 " was not generally called " zero " in English, but " nought ", which of course would make the given example futile.

I do not mean to minimise the importance of this source of error. We have to guard against it very carefully in arranging our experiments, or prove it to be inadequate to explain the results obtained. If my experiments on this point are tested, they are found to offer no evidence in favour of this explanation ; in fact, everything goes against it. Miss von B. had no notion of the kind of experiments we were going to try ; it was not a case of numbers only, where a six and a seven might have been taken for one another because of the " s ". Any other word in the whole of the German language might have been used ; we might have expected words like " brown " and " gown " to be mistaken for each other. But there is not a single case in the reports which lends support to a mistake of this type. On the other hand, it is most improbable that the whispering should have been loud enough for every single word to be heard accurately. Now, it might be assumed that Miss von B. had heard the word " violin " at the beginning of the experiment, and went to the length of making wordy descriptions of what she had seen. But we have no positive grounds for such an assumption ; everything speaks for the description of a visual perception. The same holds good for Miss S. In this case also we have no grounds for thinking that Miss S. had an auditive perception of the object. I had warned the agent, and she took particular care not to whisper ; but suppose she had unwittingly transmitted the words " Two rectangles . . . a small one . . . like the sign of the Jews . . . a rectangle . . . a small one . . . a triangle ", it is most unlikely that the agent, by means of whispers which escaped the notice of the people around her, should have transmitted so clear an impression of these figures in space, that the recipient would be able to make a special drawing. I watched the agent and know that she did not draw the figure in the air. If we tried to reproduce the drawing with closed eyes we could hardly do it better.

A critic of occultism once said that science could only recognize telepathy if the messages were transmitted from one closed room to another. Of course it would be very good if it were so, and several cases are reported in which it was done, but it is not possible to fix a priori the conditions under which phenomena are to occur if they are to be acceptable. From the methodological point of view it is as reasonable as if we were to require light to pass through metal in optical experiments instead of only through glass. It seems to me that this proof could be effected by the arrangement of the experiment in other ways. It might be theoretically impossible for a telepathic message to go through solid walls without being considerably diminished, whereas it might pass through air quite easily. The right way is to begin with experiments where agent and percipient are in the same room, and then proceed to experiments where they are in different rooms. If the latter are successful, all the better ; but the fact that they may not be cannot be taken as an exposure of the first series.

Miss von B. has strongly developed clairvoyance, as we shall see. This makes it possible that the above results are due to clairvoyance and that she may have had visions of the objects in question. In experiment No. 4 she must either have had a vision of the object when it was chosen or seen it in Wasielewski's mind. But let us consider the other experiments first. This explanation is possible, but as Wasielewski says, the clairvoyant visions are much more rapid.[1] Miss von B. seems to have the faculty of adjusting herself to these different operations.

The next point which strikes us when we consider the experiments more closely is that everything seems to suggest visual transference of the image of the object or visual conceptions of the same. These transferred images appear to emphasize details with great clearness and accuracy. For instance, Miss von B. says once : " it sparkles tremendously " ; another time she sees the strings of the violin. The transference does not seem to take the form of a rough impression of the contours, etc., of the object, but details such as the strings and the chin-rest of the violin—the " dark spot on the top of it " was recognized as the chin-rest after the experiment was over—were clearly perceived before the object was identified. I think we may consider this as a striking peculiarity if we compare it with the way in which objects appear to normal vision. If we look at an unknown object from a distance in semi-darkness,

[1] Whether this difference is due to the agent or to the percipient is not quite clear. I had an interesting case in point, where parts of rooms in a house several hundreds of miles away were described to me as I pictured them to myself ; a door I had left out being felt as a gap and seen as soon as I concentrated my mind on it. The images may have been formed by my putting the seer into direct communication with the objects themselves, as a gem would do, by my concentrating on them ; or by his actually perceiving something of the images which were forming in my mind. I had left out the door consciously, going on to the next characteristic object. [*Trans.*]

or when lit up for a very short time, we shall recognize it and be able to describe it long before we perceive such minute details. From these considerations it would seem that the recipient perceives the object in a way which could perhaps best be described by saying that he sees it through a mist in which there are gaps now and again. The fact that the agent holds in his mind during transmission a general conception or rather image of the object, which is broken by vivid flashes of this or that detail as his attention or his gaze wanders from one part of the object to the other, makes this mode of transmission probable.

It is particularly interesting that the " dark spot ", i.e. the chin-rest, should have been perceived, although Wasielewski did not transmit it consciously. This would lead us to surmise that it was due to clairvoyance, or to the transmission of visions or ideas which were not in the centre of attention or consciousness of the agent. We probably need not go so far as to say that it is due to transmission of ideas from the subconscious mind. It seems to me that the facts are covered by the transmission of details not consciously noticed, which have of course left their impress on the retina and caused the consequent changes in the brain without drawing attention to themselves. So we need not call in clairvoyance as an explanation, but we cannot exclude the possibility of its presence.

There seems to be no indication in my experiments of auditive perceptions accompanying the visual perceptions (this statement holds good only for the experiments hitherto reported, and should not be considered as a general statement). Given the right kind of experiment, agent, and recipient, with the right kind of conceptual habit, the reception of sound-perceptions or auditive conceptions should be possible.[1]

---

[1] Wasielewski transmitted tunes successfully to Miss von B. He thought of a tune, and she would begin to hum it.

EXPERIMENTS

In Kotik's experiments with his first medium, for instance, the perceptions of the medium seem to have been largely of an auditive nature ; this is not surprising, as words were being transmitted to a medium with a particularly well-developed acoustic sense.

I cannot find a single experiment which would point to the transmission having taken place by unconscious whispering. If we want to try to explain my results by the "whispering" theory, then it should be particularly obvious in experiment No. 4, where Wasielewski held Miss von B.'s hand, and they were much closer to each other than in the other experiments. But in this case the transmission was particularly bad and the experiment had to be altered. This is a strong argument against the above theory, as otherwise the course of this experiment is not surprising. Wasielewski had a mental picture of an object that he had only just seen for a very short time. The experiment proceeded normally as soon as he had the object in front of him, probably because the picture in his mind was more vivid. We can take it for granted that Miss von B. did not see the bottle ; the arrangement of the experiment made it impossible.

This is the only experiment which is at all similar to the "muscle-reading" previously discussed. In this case indications for the carrying out of some action could have been given involuntarily, but surely not the description of an object. Voluntary communications would be quite out of the question with persons like Miss von B. and Wasielewski. The only way in which transmission could have taken place effectively in this way was by some prearranged code, and this is still more ridiculous than the above supposition. It may happen that the hand of the agent draws simple objects in the air unconsciously, but this does not apply here ; the characteristic sparkling and other qualities were given before Miss von B.'s hand was held. Then she did not get any further while her hand was being held, and finally, the experiment proceeded well and quickly when the agent was looking at the object.

Some of my readers may think that I have gone out of my way to discuss the most far-fetched explanations as to how transmission might take place. But it has happened so often in occultism that a critic supposes the experimenter has neglected a source of error, or failed to realize it, because he did not discuss it at length. It is rather bold to assume that because an objection was not considered, or a possible source of error was not pointed out by the author, this particular error probably crept in. But such statements have often been made, and have had their effect, so that an uneasy feeling has remained long after the objection had been proved to be mistaken. It is therefore best to mention all these points beforehand.

The failures and difficulties met with by the medium often help to throw light on the mechanism of the faculty in action—much more so than the really successful experiments. The experiment with the flask is one of these. It gives us the impression that Miss von B. was on a wrong track. She told us afterwards that she had the fountain called the Wittelsbacher-Brunnen, in Munich, in her mind ; probably the sparkling had suggested it to her. She had seen it a few days previously and it had made a great impression on her. She followed these associations up to a certain point, but did not quite accept them. It might well have been the case that Wasielewski had a picture of this fountain before him or that he tried to call it back to memory. But she does not say " it is a fountain ", or " it is the Wittelsbacher-Brunnen ", as she said in the case of the violin or the scissors, but seems to feel that there is something wrong ; perhaps she thinks that it might be due to association, and not the object Wasielewski had in his mind. Although she is quick-witted, combination seems to play but a small part in her answers. It is also interesting to note that the size of the objects in experiments 2 and 3 are given at random, to be corrected sooner or later in the course of the experiment.

The only time when any actual help was given was when Wasielewski said : " Is it not getting larger or clearer ? " in experiment No. 3. It may be that it did actually help her, as she said " getting large " soon after, but it was meagre help, and most of the important statements were volunteered by her quite apart from this. Miss von B. says that the image of the object becomes visible quite alone, so that the determination of its size must often be difficult. When we see a thing we get an appreciation of its real size either by comparing it with known things surrounding it or by identifying it. Wasielewski's attempts to mislead her at the end of this experiment with the question : " What colour ? " and the statement : " We will only proceed with this experiment for a short time so as not to tire you, and then stop," were meant to suggest to her that she had not passed the initial stage of the experiment, but they had no effect at all ; on the contrary she stated more emphatically that what she had described was correct.

B. Clairvoyance

(a) Cryptoscopic Experiments

Dr. v. Wasielewski and I were able to have two further séances with Miss v. B. in the autumn of 1913. They were a continuation of the series we had begun in 1912. The experiments took place in my flat in Munich, and only the three of us were present. Dr. v. Wasielewski very kindly allowed me the sole publication of these experiments, only mentioning them quite briefly in his book.

TELEPATHY AND CLAIRVOYANCE

Before the arrival of Miss v. B., Wasielewski and I collected a large number of post cards from my last month's correspondence, and asked my wife to give me some also. I made a packet of them, and locked them up in my writing-table. Miss v. B. agreed to give us an experiment under definite test conditions. Mrs. Tischner, Wasielewski, and I were present.

6th Experiment. Object : a post card of unknown contents.

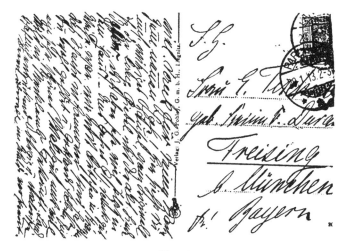

FIG. 3.

I went to my study alone, locked the door behind me, picked one of the post cards out of the packet, without looking at it, and wrapped it up in a piece of black paper, such as is used to wrap up photographic plates. I then put this packet into a thick purple-lined envelope sealing it five times with violet sealing wax, and using my seal—Dr. R. T. I locked all the things I had used in my roll-top writing table, so that no writing materials were left in the room.

42

Miss v. B. was afraid our presence might disturb her ; she said that she had not done any experiments for several months, and did not know us well. I agreed to her conditions in the hope that I would soon have an opportunity of being present at an experiment. The medium lay down on a couch and a lighted candle was put on a chair by her side ; then she was given the

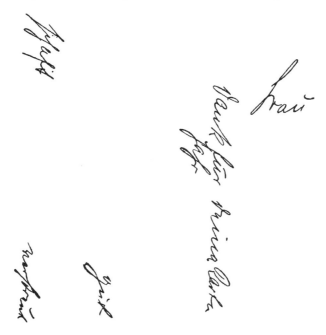

FIG. 4.

sealed envelope, a pencil and a piece of paper, after which we left the room, switching off the electric light and leaving the door ajar behind us. We all sat in the next room, I got up and peeped into the room several times without noticing anything suspicious. After about five minutes I came into the room unexpectedly, and found the medium still lying on the sofa, holding the sealed envelope to her head. She handed it to me as well as a piece of paper on which she had written a few words. The envelope seals and seams were unaltered, the envelope was not even crumpled. Miss v. B., before I opened the envelope in the presence of the others, said that she had paid particular attention to the text and neglected the picture.

On one side of the paper we found :

Frau—Dank für Deine Karte—Jahr—gut—schaft—verstreut.

Mrs.—thanks for your card—year—good—scape—strewn.

This is more clearly seen in the figure. She had written the following words on the other side of the paper :

" Picture, not a head, or animal, a house between trees, but not quite certain, a plain house."

As can be seen in figure 5, the picture could hardly be better described than by the words : " A plain

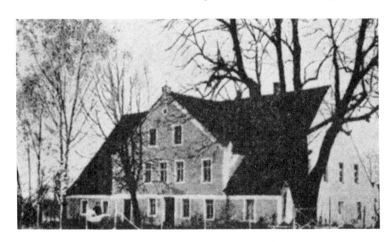

Fig. 5.

44

house between trees." On the written side of the card only a few words had been read, but these quite correctly, and placed in exactly the same positions as on the original. It would hardly have been possible to place them better if they were being copied. We will discuss the writing later, but the single syllable " schaft " of the word " landschaftlich " is interesting.

SITTING NEXT EVENING

Present : the same people as on the previous evening, the late occultist, Dr. Walter Bormann, and Privatdozent Dr. med. Franz Schede.

7th Experiment. Object : an unknown post card.

I handed a packet of about 300 to 400 picture post cards, which had been tied up in a bundle and not looked at for years, to Dr. Bormann and Dr. Schede, so that they should make similar preparations to those of the previous evening. I put black paper, an envelope, sealing-wax, and a seal at their disposal ; then Wasielewski, my wife, and I left the room. Dr. Schede pulled a card out of the packet and handed it to Dr. Bormann, who wrapped it up in black paper, and put this into an envelope, which he proceeded to close and sealed five times. I came back when they had finished, and locked up all they had used in the writing table, before leading Miss v. B. into the room. She lay down on the sofa ; I handed her the envelope, paper, and a pencil, lighted the candle and left her, just as on the previous evening. I looked several times through the crack of the slightly open door and saw nothing which could possibly arouse my suspicion ; after about five minutes I went into the room and took the envelope from her, we all examined it, and found it unchanged.

Before I opened the envelope Miss v. B. said :
" The first word of the address is " Family ".

When I heard this, I must say, I thought that the experiment was a failure, and that the data were drawn from her imagination; I could not remember ever receiving a card addressed " Family Dr. Tischner ". Such a mode of addressing letters would be most unlikely. " Family " was the only word read on this

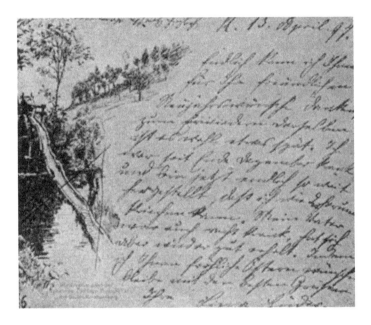

FIG. 6.

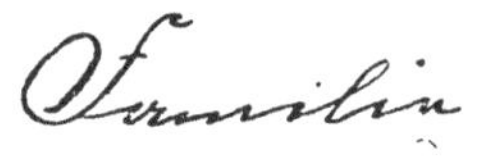

FIG. 6a (Original).

side of the card. The following words were scattered on the other side :

" Endlich kann—jetzt—Mein Vater—Lina Luder."

" Can at last—now—My father—Lina Luder."

and there was the beginning of a drawing. Miss v. B.

46

explained that there was a picture on the other side of the card which was not separated from the text in the usual way, but which ran into the text, as it were. She had seen two main lines of this picture, and had drawn them.

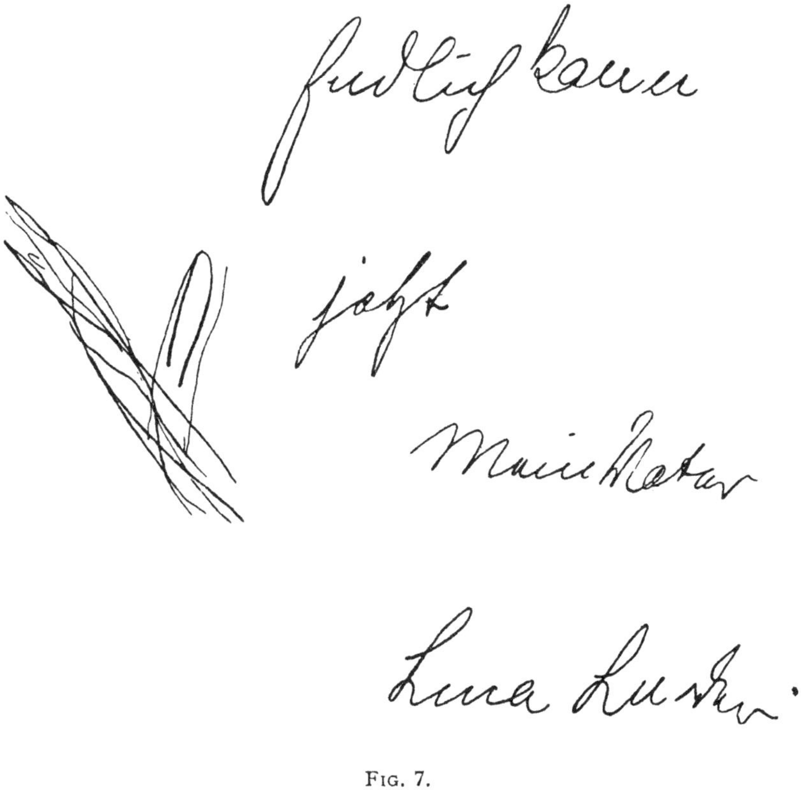

FIG. 7.

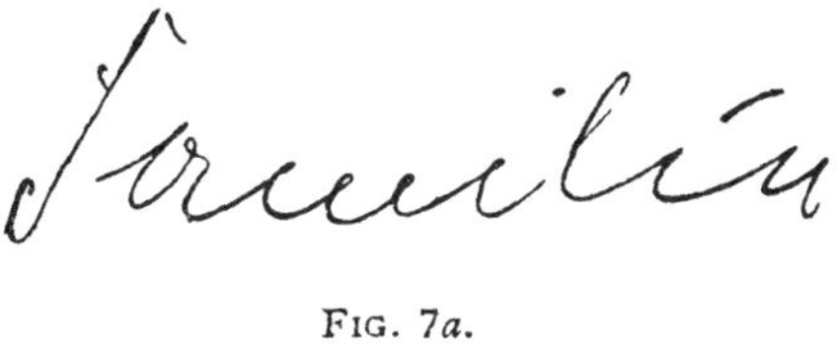

FIG. 7a.

When we opened the envelope we found that the first word of the address was the word " Family ". The card had been written to my father's family in 1897 by a chance acquaintance made at a watering place. So the card was 16½ years old, and I should hardly be likely to have read it again, as it came from a casual acquaintance. There really was a drawing on the same side as the text, the two main lines drawn were correct, and the picture was not separated from the text by the usual line. Both the words and their places in the text were correct, the only mistake being rather a characteristic one. The signature was written " Luder " instead of "Lüder", a slip which would have been noticed on reflection, as the surname Luder [1] would certainly be very rare if it exists at all. (See Figs. 6, 6a, 7, 7a.)

8th Experiment. Object : a small cardboard box containing cotton wool. The contents were unknown to us.

The next experiment that evening was planned as follows : I wanted to try an experiment similar to Wasielewski's with small boxes, but we had not got a number of absolutely similar ones. So Mrs. Tischner and I each fetched a small box out of our jewel-cases, without looking at the contents. These we handed to Dr. Bormann and Dr. Schede, leaving it to them to choose one, after we had left the room. They packed the chosen box in black paper, put it in an envelope, and sealed it ; it was then handed to Miss v. B. who lay down on the sofa and tried to visualize the contents. Mrs. Tischner and Dr. Schede were in the room all the time, the former writing down word for word what the medium said.

" A feeling as if it were nothing, and yet something— not hollow but not full either—feels like feathers. Nothing and yet something, very light, shapeless, but like a sponge-finger, filled with something—a disagreeable feeling—it is scarcely coloured at all."

---

[1] "Luder" means rascal. [*Trans.*]

EXPERIMENTS

Miss v. B. said that the experiment tired her very much, so that she nearly felt faint and was inclined to give it up as a failure. On opening the box we found a piece of cotton-wool about $3\frac{1}{8}$ ins. by $\frac{3}{4}$ in. by $\frac{1}{2}$ in. The object itself was not named, but was so pregnantly described : " Nothing and yet something—it is not hollow, but it is not full either—very light and shapeless —like feathers " ; that we can consider the experiment as a complete success, although not so striking as the recognition of a word at a definite place on a page, with all the characteristics of the original writing. *Positive.*

I stayed at the medium's house in June, 1916, and had hoped to continue our series of experiments. Miss v. B. had married in the interval, and had apparently lost all her psychic power through neglect. As we expected, she was not able to read a note in a sealed envelope ; I shall not include this experiment, as there was nothing supernormal in it owing to the lack of mediumistic power.

SITTING WITH MISS S.

9th Experiment. Object : a known short note in a lined envelope.

This experiment was tried with Miss S. at her first table-turning séance in my rooms. She nearly fell into trance several times during the séance, so I finally put her into trance by an order and a few passes. I handed her a lined envelope containing a short note I had written some time ago ; I picked this note from several without looking to see which one it was. She very soon said :

" Wednesday past (pause, I gave her an energetic order to go on) child—pain."

On opening the note we found :

" It is Thursday to-day."

At first I did not pay any particular attention to this, in fact I hardly noticed it, regarding the experiment as

49

a failure, till someone said : " Wednesday past is Thursday." We often find such semi-exact results in the English accounts of automatic writing, in Mrs. Verrall's for instance. So we can look at this experiment in a different light. There certainly is a danger of reading meanings into these statements. In some cases I for my part hold that this has been done. So I leave it to my critics to pass a verdict on this experiment. I just wanted to mention it in connexion with the English cases. The day on which the experiment was made was a Friday, so the day mentioned on the paper did not correspond with it, but I will not go so far as to maintain that the medium spoke in such general terms to avoid making a definitely false statement ; this would hardly be consistent with the psychology of hypnotism.

We will pass on to a series of experiments with a third medium.

On the afternoon of 18th May, 1918, Mr. R., who is in touch with occult circles, came to me with a Mr. Re, who said he was a clairvoyant. Mr. Re had come to him and had gone through several tests successfully, so he had come to me at once, knowing that for years I had been looking for a clairvoyant.

Mr. Re was 32, and his father was a post office official in Munich. I gathered from his papers that he had been sent back from the front in 1916 to an auxiliary hospital for a few months suffering from hysteria. He said that he was feeling quite well now. He told me that he had often done legerdemain tricks for a small circle, and among other things, clairvoyance. He had discovered this faculty by chance a few years ago. In his performances he used to read the contents of small folded slips in the following way. He would fail to read the first, open it, and look at it, but not read the contents aloud. He then took up the second slip, stated the contents of the first slip, opened the second slip, said the answer was correct, and remembered the contents of the second for the third. Of course, he had to prevent anyone from actually checking the readings ; the supposed confirmation of the accuracy of his readings was that whenever he read a slip one of the spectators claimed to have written it, and said it was quite correct. He still gives performances.

We must consider him as decidedly suspect, and great care must be taken to prevent any fraud, especially as Re was quite without means at the time, and this was his only means of earning his living.

There are two kinds of critics of occultism. The one class says that paid mediums are unreliable, owing to the fact that they are paid and therefore are dependent on the apparent success of their experiments ; the others say that unpaid mediums are suspect because you cannot enforce test conditions to the same extent as with a paid medium, especially as the medium is generally a lady, and the experimenters are inclined to credulity and indulgence. I am in the fortunate, or perhaps unfortunate, position of having spoilt my case with both sides, as Miss v. B. and Miss S. are unpaid mediums, and Mr. Re is a paid medium. *Incidit in Scyllam qui vult evitare Charybdin.* So it will be impossible to hope for unanimity of opinion, as one group will object to the one series of experiments and the other to the other. I can only live in hopes that there may be a third group who can appreciate positive data quite apart from conditions which might hypothetically arouse suspicion.

Mr. Re is really open to suspicion, so I have gradually enforced my methods of experimentation and caused him to give up a great many of his habitual conditions, but have done so without changing the routine of his experiments. We must not forget that the methods of occultism vary tremendously with their object. In dark sittings it is very difficult to have strictly test conditions, and it is not easy to get rid of the feeling that one might be deceived, especially when dealing with a paid medium, whose chief object must be to produce phenomena. In dealing with clairvoyance the conditions are quite different, and more transparent from the very first. I have tried to make them as clear and simple as possible for absent critics by reducing the action and making it take place solely between the medium and the experimenter. This gives a kind of cinematographic picture of the whole proceedings in which it is possible to follow every movement. Unfortunately I was often prevented from carrying out my plan by the medium asking for slips written by others present, so as to get into contact with them. I cannot judge whether he was justified in doing so or not.

The Whitsuntide holidays and a series of unfortunate coincidences prevented my being able to secure the presence of one of the philosophers or psychologists of the university, although I tried very hard to do so, and Re had to leave Munich soon after, being judged fit for army service. The general conditions of the experiments in the summer of 1918 were as follows : I wrote down the few words he said during the experiment, keeping an eye on him all the while, or in the intervals between the experiments ; I generally sat a yard or two from him, but several times I stood by his side in a very well-lighted room, so that I could watch every movement and would certainly have detected any attempt on his part to look at a sign or number on the outside of the slip.

I wanted to test his powers by handing him one of my specially prepared envelopes, but he refused it, saying that he was used to small slips folded three times. To avoid putting him off at the start, I prepared a few slips about $\frac{3}{4}$ of an inch by 1 inch. Re stood with his back to me watched by Mr. R., while I stood 15–17 ft.

EXPERIMENTS

from him and wrote several slips with a soft pencil, rubbing the back of the slip with my thumb-nail every time, then folding it three times, making the fold in the middle of the long side every time, so that each fold was at right angles to the previous one and the folded slip similar to a postage stamp in shape and about half its size. I knew Hennig's paper on the possible tricks used in reading slips, having recently reviewed it, so I took all the necessary precautions to prevent Re from practising any of them. I did not give Re a chance of seeing the writing-pad at a distance of less than 9 feet, and always locked it up in my desk immediately after writing. I mixed the slips several times and threw them up into the air, thus obviating sources of error due to my knowing the contents of the slip. Mr. R. also wrote some slips, using his pocket-book as a pad—and putting it back into his pocket as soon as he had finished writing : I watched Re carefully all the time.

Re generally holds the slips between thumb and index finger, but he sometimes holds them in the hollow of his hand, with arm stretched out horizontally to one side or obliquely in front of him. It is rarely that he holds a slip to his forehead, in fact, he mostly turns his head away from the hand holding the slip and avoids looking in that direction. He will try holding the slip in the other hand if the visualization is long in coming ; this he may repeat several times, but there is nothing suspicious about the procedure, the change of hands being effected quite low down, not level with his face. He often has twitchings in the cervical muscle and in the muscle of the arm.

Re said he did not like making experiments in the afternoon ; he much preferred the evening, as they were decidedly more successful. Still, I picked up one of the slips which lay on the table and handed it to him.

TELEPATHY AND CLAIRVOYANCE

SITTING OF 18TH MAY, 1918

10*th Experiment.* Object : a slip containing the Russian words " Ja nje ponimaju " in Roman type.

After trying unsuccessfully for about half a minute to make out what was on the slip he asked me whether I had written single disconnected syllables. He said he could not read them.

I asked for the slip, opened it, and found that I had written the above Russian words. Re explained that he did not mean to say that the syllables were disconnected in space, but that they made no sense for him taken collectively. He knew that I had written the slip. So he was not quite wrong. *Doubtful.*

11*th Experiment.* Object : a slip containing the Italian sentence " Io anche pittore ".

Re was not able to read this slip : he stuck at the first letters. He said : " I can't read the first letters."

He got no further. I was in a hurry when writing, so that the letters were rather peculiarly shaped and difficult to read, a fact which would tell more in a foreign language. *Negative*, with extenuating circumstances.

12*th Experiment.* Object : a slip containing the number 26.

" This slip is written by R.   It contains the number 26." *Positive.*

13*th Experiment.* Object : a slip with the number 100.

" Also written by Mr. R.—it has three digits—100." *Positive.*

14*th Experiment.* Object : a slip inscribed with " Athens is the capital of Greece ".

He said at once : " A sentence in German—but I can't read all of it—the first word is ' Athens '."

He got no further. I encouraged him to go on reading and said that the writing was probably rather illegible ;

he said he did not think that that mattered, but it was due to the fact that he was not so well disposed in the daytime as in the evening. So I opened the slip. We cannot consider this experiment negative, for it is not possible to guess the word " Athens ". *Positive.*

15th Experiment. Object : a slip with the word " Sebald ".

Re said very quickly : " Mr. R.'s—Sebald." *Positive.*

I then tried a few psychoscopic (psychometric) experiments—not here recorded—without success.

SITTING OF THE SAME EVENING

When R. and Re had arrived, I adjourned to the next room and wrote five slips. R. watched Re the while, and I left the writing-pad in the room where I had written, a room Re did not enter. Then R. went and wrote five slips while I watched Re. The ten slips were folded up, well mixed and put on the table. On this occasion, as in the afternoon, we both used the same paper, so that it was impossible to tell from the outside which of us had written any given slip. I said that before the beginning of the experiments I had written five numbers, and each containing 3 digits. As R. said that Re's powers were more telepathic than clairvoyant, I had written my five numbers on a slip and looked at them several times during the course of the experiments. This enabled me to say that the figures 337 and 367 in experiment No. 19 were wrong. It is obvious that his knowledge of the figures did not enable him to tell the number on the slip held in his hand. The clairvoyant with whom Schottelius experimented also stated that his powers inclined towards telepathy. This gave me the impression that he had been induced to make this statement under the influence of suggestive questions or that it was to his interest to deny his faculty. A police official told me subsequently that clairvoyance was punishable as a form of charlatanism, whereas telepathy was not. This explains the otherwise ridiculous statements of Re and Kahn.

Re sometimes picked out single slips himself in this sitting, but as he always handed them to me unopened as soon as he had spoken, exchange seems impossible.[1]

16th Experiment. Object : a slip inscribed with the word " Absollon ".

After about 10 seconds Re said : " ' Abholen ' is written on the slip."

We opened the slip and found the above. R. explained that he had meant to write Absalom, and had not remembered how to spell it. It is very easy to mistake the long Germanic s for an h. *Positive* in the main features.

17th Experiment. Object: a slip with the number 434. " A number with three digits—434." *Positive.*

18th Experiment. Object : a slip with the number 231.

"Again Dr. Tischner's—three digits—231." *Positive.*

19th Experiment. Object: a slip with the number 987. " Again a number with three digits—337— (T. : ' No ')—367—(T. : ' No ')—but there is a 7 at the end."

The last figure and the rounded character of the figures had been recognized. *Positive,* in part.

20th Experiment. Object : a slip with " Eberhard " on it. Written by Mr. R. Eberhard.

I asked him to write down the word as nearly like the original as possible. The similarity is striking. *Positive.*

21st Experiment. Object : a slip with the number 521.

---

[1] The author does not think there could have been double substitution, but of course it was not impossible at this sitting. [*Trans.*]

He said at once, " It is written by Dr. T."

Then he took a pencil and wrote down "521" without saying a word. I asked him whether he always made a dot over his " 1 ". He said quite decidedly : " No, but you have made one."

This was before we opened the slip. *Positive.*

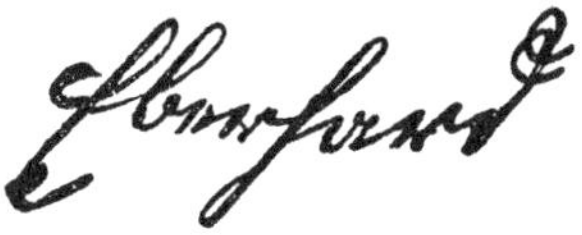

FIG. 8. 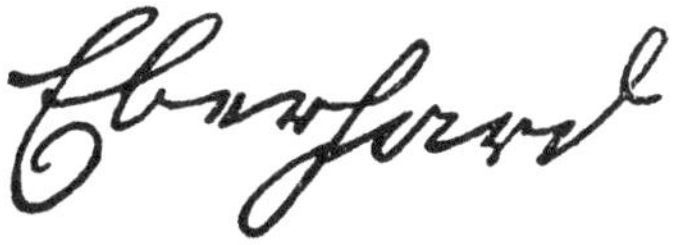 FIG. 9 (Original).

22nd Experiment. Object : a slip with " München " on it. " By Mr. R—vague—München."

I asked him to write it out, which he did. It was in Roman type, whereas Eberhard was in German type ; he had recognized both. *Positive.*

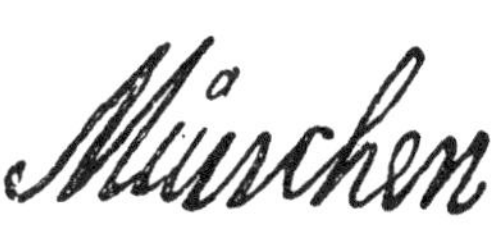

FIG. 10. 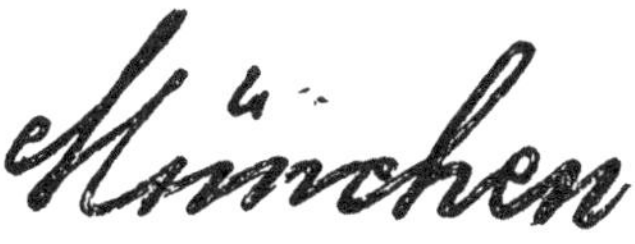 FIG. 11 (Original).

23rd Experiment. Object: a slip with the number 777. " Not at all clear—Mr. R., have you written a number ? "—(R. " Yes ")—" You have not made a full stop, so I don't know whether it is 666 or 999." On opening it we found 777 written by me.

24th Experiment. Object : a slip with 666 or 999. " The same number." *Positive.*

25th Experiment. Object : a slip with the word " Faust ".

" One word—Faust." *Positive.*

SITTING OF 20TH MAY AT 3.30 P.M.

Re appeared unexpectedly on Whit-Monday at 3.30 p.m. with the intention of putting off the sitting that evening ; he subsequently decided to stay.

He rejected a number of slips I had prepared, saying they were too large for him, as he was used to smaller ones. A great many people have their peculiarities when doing intellectual work, some have to chew a penholder, some to smell rotten apples, etc., so I conceded the point. I wrote four small slips while he was standing in the hall, folded three times like the previous ones, and put them in my pocket. I then darkened the room slightly by drawing the curtains, which were thin. A Miss J. was present besides Re and myself.

26th Experiment. Object: slip with " Wer nie sein Brot mit Tränen as." [1]

He tried in vain to read the first slip. I asked him to give it back to me, which he did, saying that he was in much better form in the evening. Consequently, I suggested that we should adjourn to the next room, which I could darken completely, and try again by artificial light. He said that he did not think that it was the light but the time of day which affected him, but he agreed to try all the same. So we went into the next room ; I switched on the light, let down the blind and handed him the slip which I had kept in a separate pocket. Progress was slow.

" Not many words—the words in three lines— Roman type—is there a word ' Brand ' in it ?—At any rate there is a capital ' B ' in Roman type, then an ' r ', it finishes up with a hard ' t ' and there are two letters in between. Perhaps it is ' Braut '. —(T. : ' You have got on the wrong track, you seem to have come to a dead stop ')—Aha ! you mean the two letters—I see quite short words—there is not a single long word among them. It is not ' Brett '—' Brot '—I think it is ' Brot '. It seems to be a quotation."

---

[1] " Who never eats his bread with tears " (Goethe). [*Trans.*]

We broke off the experiment, so as to take it up again later. I particularly want to emphasize that I realized which slip he had in his hand as soon as he said that the first word was " Brand " and then more emphatically that it began with " Br " and ended with " t ". I had had no notion which one he had got before then, and did not think of any one particular slip.

As a matter of fact we did not repeat this experiment. But " Brot " and the fact that it was a quotation were correct ; also the statement that it consisted of three lines written in Roman type. Before unfolding the slip we asked him more details about it. He said that he had noticed this from the accentuation.

He probably meant " rhythm ". *Positive.*

27th Experiment. Object : slip with " Barbara " on it.

" Only one word—veiled—begins with a ' B '—second later ' a ' or ' o '—' a '—' Barbar '—' Barbara '."

I had forgotten this word altogether, I was not even clearly conscious of it when he said " Barbar ". *Positive.*

28th Experiment. Object : slip with the number " 21244 ".

" Seems to be one word—I see a capital ' A ' as the first letter, but this is not correct."

On being asked for more details about his last remark, he said that it did not fit into the picture produced by the whole word. We broke off the experiment, as he did not seem to be able to get on any further.

29th Experiment. Object : slip with " Agathe " on it.

" An ' A '—again a name like Barbara—' Alfred '—' Agathe '. *Positive.*

28th Experiment (continued).

" Seems to be a number—I see a number—the second digit is your characteristic ' 1 '—it has five digits—I can't read the third—the first is a ' 2 '—' twenty-one

thousand '—' two hundred '—twice the same figure—
' 44 '—' 21244 '." *Positive.*

I knew what was on the slip in both these last
experiments. I asked him to write down the number,
which he did. He put a dot on the ' 1 '. I could not
remember whether I had done so, but we subsequently
found that I had not done so. I asked him to rewrite
the two " 4's ", which he did, putting in the two loops
I had purposely made at the corners, and which he had
omitted the first time.

SITTING OF 20TH MAY AT 8.30 P.M.

Present : Mrs. J., Miss T., Mrs. Tischner, Re, and
myself. I had written a number of slips with a soft
lead pencil before the sitting, and folded them three
times in the usual way. I now chose four of these and
put them in the right-hand pocket of my coat. I
particularly wanted to prevent Re from having any
influence whatever on the sequence and management
of the experiments. I handed the slips to Re ; the
experiments went very quickly, so that in experiments
30–32 Re held the slips in his left hand with his arm
stretched out horizontally and his head turned to the
right all the time. I took the slip away from him as
soon as he had finished his answer, and opened it
myself. So it was quite impossible for him to exchange
any of the slips in this series. At the end of the
experiment four of the slips I had written lay before
me on the table.

30*th Experiment.* Object : slip with the words
" Happy is the man who can shut himself up from the
world without hatred."

" Short—not long."

He was unable to say more, so I took away the slip
after eight minutes, and put it into another pocket.

31*st Experiment.* Object : slip with the word
" Freising ".

EXPERIMENTS

" One word—Tr, no—Frei, no—Freising."

The experiment went very quickly, he made the first statement after 8 or 10 seconds, and had finished the experiment after 30–40 seconds. *Positive.*

32nd Experiment. Object : slip with the word " Mandoline ".

" Vague — one single word — Madeline, no — Mandoline."

This took three quarters of a minute. I asked him to write down the word with all the peculiarities of my writing ; the " M " and the " d " were not like the originals, the other letters were less liable to be written differently from mine. *Positive.*

33rd Experiment. Object : slip with a drawing.

" Very strange—not a word—not a number. Have you made a drawing, Dr. Tischner ? "

He drew what he saw. The most prominent features were correct. *Positive.*

  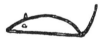

Fig. 12.   Fig. 13 (Original).

30th Experiment (continued).

" I can see nothing." *Negative.*

I took five slips written in ink that afternoon out of the writing-table, and handed one of them to him.

34th Experiment. Object : slip with the word " Helsingfors ".

" I don't perceive anything." *Negative.*

Sitting of 22nd May

I include here the report of the sitting of 22nd May,[1] although a large circle brings disturb-

---

[1] Tischner answers a critic : " I regard these experiments as inferior, and only include them for the sake of completeness. Other critics have thanked me for doing so (*Monistische Monatsblätter*, 1921). [*Trans.*]

ing factors with it and influences which can be avoided in small sittings. I had the control of the sitting, and the experiments were carried on in much the same way as before. Re distributed a number of small slips of paper, asking the audience to write something on them and to fold them three times. He then collected the slips. Twenty-one persons had written slips, and twenty-one slips lay before me on the table. Mostly I handed Re the slip ; sometimes he took one up himself. At the end of each experiment he handed the folded slip to me. He generally made use of the pauses to go out and have a breath of fresh air, as it was oppressively hot in the room.

35th Experiment. Object : slip with the word " Madelene ".

" Roman type—the word is not correct—it is either misspelt or vague—Has anyone written Madalene ? " *Positive.*

36th Experiment. Object : slip with the word " Arturo ".

He does not perceive anything, and gives it up. The word was written in very thin and illegible handwriting. *Negative.*

37th Experiment. Object : slip with the name " Carmen ".

" A name—not a German name—C, very large, very small writing—seems to have been written by a lady—Carmen."

Actually it was written by a lady. He wrote it down as he saw it and hit off the character of the writing very well, with the exception of the " C ". *Positive.*

38th Experiment. Object : slip with " Panta re " in Roman type.

" Seems to be French, very small writing, perhaps : ' vive le roi '—at any rate ' roi ' or ' rei '—three words or three syllables—' Panta rei '." *Positive.*

39*th Experiment.* Object : slip with " Ludwig Wilser " and a few sanscrit letters.

" Not at all clear—a gentleman has written it—two words—with cabalistic signs or something of that sort under them—' Ludwig Wilser '."

He wrote down the sanscrit letters as he saw them. The first is very good. *Positive.*

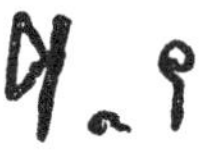

FIG. 14.

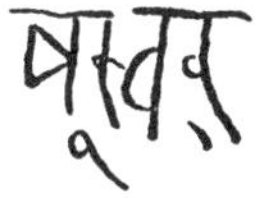

FIG. 15 (Original).

40*th Experiment.* Object : slip with the name ' Frommert.'

" Only one word—at most five letters or four— ' Anna ' or ' Unna '." *Negative.*

41*st Experiment.* Object : slip with " Zacharias ".

" Very well written—a name—begins with a ' Z '— ' Zacharias '." *Positive.*

42*nd Experiment.* Object : slip with " Sarastro ".

" Quite a foreign name—very well written, Zoroa, no—Zarathust, no—Zarastro." Practically correct. *Positive.*

43*rd Experiment.* Object : slip with " Cannstadt ".

" Curious, the first letter is a ' C '—' Stadt '— ' Cannstadt '."

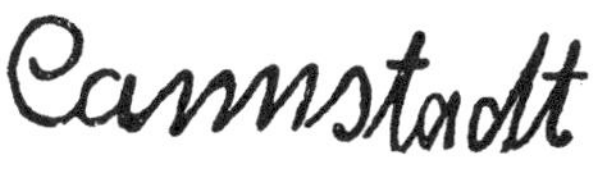

FIG. 16.

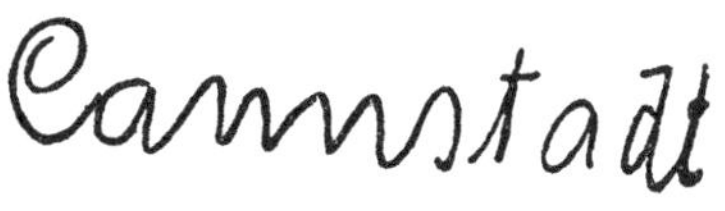

FIG. 17 (Original).

He writes the name as he sees it, quite correctly, but with a ' dt ' at the end. As it turned out, the lady who had written the slip had written Cannstadt instead of Cannstatt, to mislead him. *Positive.*

44th Experiment. Object : slip with " Pater ".
" Difficult—Roman type, Latin—very well written
—' Pater '." *Positive.*
After a long absence, Re came back to Munich. It
was in February, 1919. He came to see me and agreed
to hold a sitting on the 8th at 8 p.m.

I prepared a number of slips ; on twelve of these I
wrote figures with three digits, placing the figures to
the left of and above the centre of the slip, so that the
figure should be on a flat surface when the slip was
folded. Hitherto, I had found it quite immaterial
whether the writing was overlapping or not, but I
wanted to make the task as easy as possible. I folded
eight of them once and then carefully stuck the edges
with gum ; then I went on to fold them in the usual
way. By placing the writing as I had done, I had
arranged it in the middle of the slip with three thicknesses of paper on one side and four on the other.
The remaining four were left ungummed. I wrote
words of figures, or made a drawing, on three more
slips which I gummed. I put these three different
kinds of slips in different pockets.

SITTING OF 8TH FEBRUARY, 1919, AT 8 P.M.

Present : Dr. med. F. Schede, *privatdozent* at the
University of Munich, Dr. Paul Flaskämper, Re and I.
We sat at about three or five feet from Re. There
were twelve other people in the room, but they acted
as spectators only, and their chairs were placed along
the opposite wall of the room, which was a large one.
I wanted these experiments to give the reader an almost
cinematographic view of the proceedings. I was to
take one step forward, hand the slip to the medium, and
then take it away from him as soon as he had finished
speaking. These were the only actions which were to
take place. The results were so poor that we were not

able to carry out this plan. I will only describe the experiments in which he was able to say something about the contents of the slip, so that I opened it. When he only gave one digit I put the slip on one side for use another time. Dr. Flaskämper kept the record.

45th Experiment. Object : gummed slip with the number " 824 ".

He took the slip in his left hand : " Letters—there seem to be letters—six or seven letters as it were in a mist—I see all through a veil." *Negative.*

46th–49th Experiments. Negative. He could say nothing.

Re said that he had not got into contact with us, and asked for a few slips written by other people. After making a few objections I agreed to do so. I handed four slips to four ladies, collected them as soon as they were written, and gave one to Re.

50th Experiment. Object : slip inscribed with " Julius ".

After a long pause : " It is quite short—but I feel that I shall succeed to-day."

Then a pause ensued in which I took the slip. I handed it back to Re. " Very neatly written—quite fine letters—one word, the first letter is ' i '— ' in '— no—I think it will go now—' Julius '. I can't make it anything else." *Positive.*

He held the slip in his left hand and was looking obliquely to the right all the time. There was nothing that could make us think that he had gained information by a trick or had tried to do so.

51st–58th Experiments. Negative.

He did not make any movement which might lead us to believe that he tried to find out the contents by fraudulent means. Dr. Schede and Dr. Flaskämper both were convinced that this was a genuine case of clairvoyance and that fraud was not possible under the circumstances, although only one experiment had been successful. These were the first supernormal phenomena of the kind witnessed by Dr. Flaskämper.

During the sitting Re kept on saying that he was quite out of practice and that a carbuncle on his neck caused him pain when he twitched and prevented success. This he repeated several times after the experiments.

SITTING ON 12TH FEBRUARY, 1919

Present: Dr. O. Schlegel, Mrs. Tischner, three other ladies, Re, and myself.

The experimental conditions were the same. The three ladies sat in the background. Mrs. Tischner kept the record.

59th-63rd Experiments. Negative.

I handed four slips to the ladies, collected them and handed them to him one by one. The next experiment is negative, but is worth mentioning as it bears a close analogy to Kotik's experiments with " thought-laden paper " in its result.

64th Experiment. Object : slip with the number 54.

" As if connected with medicine—seems to be a word in a foreign language."

As he was not able to say any more I opened the slip. It contained the number 54. I said it had nothing to do with medicine ; whereupon the lady who had written it, exclaimed : " Yes ! It is connected with medicine. When I was thinking what to write, I thought of a psychiatrist, a good friend of mine who would have been 54 had he been living." I merely mention this without laying any stress on it. (See pp. 49, 50.)

65th Experiment. Object : slip with 844 on it.

" 300—no, that is not right."

Writes down numbers 2—3—7, but says at once : " No ! I can't see it." *Negative.*

66th and *67th Experiments. Negative:*

68th Experiment. Object : slip with the number 318.
" A number—a ' 1 ' with a dot on it."
It is quite within the range of probability that the one with a dot on it should have been right. *Negative.*

The whole sitting was negative, and yet the control of the experiments was not so strict as in the previous sittings.

We felt that we must exercise Re's powers, as they had almost disappeared through disuse. I made him try automatic writing on the 15th ; he was able to do it very soon ; so I tried whether the solution could be elicited in this way, without coming into his consciousness at all. The slips used had been written by some one else.

69th Experiment. Object : a slip with : " To love is to suffer."

He soon writes :—" $a^2 + b^2 = c^2$—place in the neighbourhood—through woods." *Negative.*

70th Experiment. Object : slip with the number 18437.
He makes illegible signs. *Negative.*

Sitting of 13th June, 1919

He had come to see me by chance, and we were quite alone.

71st Experiment. Negative.

72nd Experiment. Object : a slip with 504 on it.
" A number with five digits." *Negative.*

73rd Experiment. Object : a slip with the word " Bern ".

" Again a number—there seems to be a ' 3 ' or an ' 8 ' and a ' 1'. The capital ' B ' looks rather like a ' 1 ' and a ' 3 '."

The result seems quite wrong. If, however, we do not consider the sense, but the sensuous impression instead, i.e. the direct impression given by the lines on the paper, then the result appears in a new light. The big Roman " B " looked exactly like " 13 ". The " 1 " was formed by the first thick line, the " 3 " by the two semicircles. These were only joined to the thick lines by a very fine line going from its foot to the top of the upper semicircle. Re's interpretation is quite natural, as he was expecting numbers. Experiment No. 28 shows us that he does not see the figures in their proper order, hence the fact that he begins by mentioning a " 3 " and an " 8 ". He seems to realize that there is more on the slip, as he says that a " 3 " or an " 8 " and a " 1 " are among the figures (" dabei "). So that if we judge this experiment according to the visual impression we must consider it successful, as the " 13 " became a " B " because it stood in front of other signs and letters, which Re could not make out. *Positive, in part.*

74th Experiment. Object : a slip with 934.

I told him it was probably a number with three digits, as I had hardly written any words.

" A number with three digits—907 ?—987 ?—There seems to be a ' 9 '."

Partly correct, he suspected an angular number at one end and a round one at the other. *Partly correct.*

Sitting of 20th February at Twelve

Present : Mr. Gerhart Kuttner, a medical student, who kept the record, Re and I. We sat about 3 ft. from the medium.

75th Experiment. Object : A slip with the number " 379 ".

" Seems to be a word—Geist—Seele—Gemüt [1]— a capital ' S ' or ' L '." *Negative.*

76th Experiment. Object : a slip containing the word " Carmen ".

This slip was written by the lady who had written the name " Julius " in a previous sitting. I told him this as he laid such weight on being in contact with or

[1] In English " Spirit—Soul—Mind." [*Trans.*]

attuned to the writer ; he had lost confidence in his powers, so I also told him that the slip contained only one word : knowing that this lady only wrote single words. I asked him to tell us all the ideas which came into his mind, as it is often not possible to read the words themselves, but images or perceptions connected with the word come into one's mind.

" The loneliness of the woods—mood of the forest— the soughing of boughs—a ring."

He was standing just in front of us during this experiment. *Negative.*

77th Experiment. Object : a black envelope closed with several gummed strips, containing a larger slip with the number 821 written in figures a quarter of an inch high.

I told him that the envelope contained a number with three digits. He was sitting on a chair ; first he held the envelope to his head with his left hand, then he took it in his right hand which hung loosely at his side.

" There seems to be an ' 8 ' in it—8—1—3 ? 3—1 —8 ? 1—8—3 ? This is really guesswork."

He had given two digits quite correctly : this could not be put down to chance. The envelope was seen to be unaltered before opening. *Partly positive.*

78th Experiment. Object : a small gummed slip with the word " Planegg ".

" Seems to be a number again. A 1 with a dot, and a 6 or a 9." I mentioned that the slip was written by a lady and contained one word, but he gave it up. *Negative.*

I was not able to continue my experiments with Re owing to his death, which took place recently ; and I was consequently unable to gain the interest of the university professors in this subject by letting them be present at the sittings. This was not due to lack of efforts on my part, but my experience was often similar to that recorded by William James, and referred to above. Moreover, a great many of these gentlemen were at the Front, and there were other unfavourable circumstances.

(b) Psychoscopic (Psychometric) Experiments

Psychometry is the name of the faculty possessed by certain mediums of obtaining supernormally the knowledge of events and scenes connected with objects with which they are in contact or relation, or of the owners or other people connected with these objects. These descriptions may refer to the past, present, or future; they often deal with the surroundings, or again the character and feelings of the owner or people associated with him, or the object. They consist often of mixtures of clairvoyance in space, visions of the past, what used to be called " soul-reading " and telepathic influences.

The word " psychometry " was introduced by Professor Buchanan, an American doctor who lived in the forties of last century. It is rather an unfortunate word, as nothing whatsoever is measured and no quantitative relations of any kind are dealt with. This led me to suggest the term *psychoscopy* instead ; it resembles psychometry closely enough in sound to call up the correct association, and suggests what really takes place, describing, as it were, a vision of the " soul of the object " and of its fate.

The following pages contain an account of the first series of scientifically conducted experiments on psychoscopy yet published in Germany, though there have been accounts of similar cases in America, France, and England.

But just a few remarks before going on to the reports. Traditional scientific psychology, as we find it in textbooks and scientific journals, knows next to nothing of occultism. Phenomena such as psychoscopy are regarded with the utmost suspicion as mystical and thoroughly unscientific. But it is rash to pronounce judgment on the subject without both practical and theoretical knowledge. These experiments do not generally proceed as smoothly as the traditional experiments in clairvoyance ; statements are often made which it is impossible to check, or which are false. But is this a reason for refusing to recognize these experiments ? I think it must be acknowledged that some of the statements are not explicable by chance or by guesswork, and point directly to a supernormal source. There is hardly an object whose history is known to us in all its details, so that all statements made about it may be checked. It may happen that a statement which was first thought wrong and impossible to check turns out unexpectedly to be correct. We .cannot, therefore, consider statements which we cannot check as necessarily wrong. Mr. H. saw a number of the objects by clairvoyance ; in other experiments telepathy seems to have come into play ; but as all these experiments form a series, I have not divided them up into these categories.

As remarked above, these experiments do not give such exact results as good experiments in clairvoyance, and one might be inclined to doubt their scientific value. But anyone who knows the English and American literature on the subject, will remember that there are a number of mediums who have obtained most valuable results by automatic writing, crystal-gazing, and psychometry, but in these cases also, true and false statements were all mixed up. However, the true statements were so numerous and so striking that they could not be put down to chance. This led scientific men like William James, Sidgwick, Sir Oliver Lodge, and others to regard such results as intensely valuable proofs of supernormal faculty.

This fact gives additional charm to these experiments and may increase their value, as it is possible that these phenomena may help us one day to understand the workings of these faculties ; these very false or ambiguous statements may lead us to the right explanation. There is a danger that we may give our imaginations too much free play, and this has probably been the case fairly often ; but it does not lessen the value of this class of experiments. I shall mention all the facts I know which may be taken as positive corroboration of the statements made, without committing myself to a final judgment in every case. My critics will judge these cases differently, as in many cases the exact data cannot be collected. I repeat that I do not wish it to be understood that I consider all the facts adduced by way of corroboration and commentary on an experiment, as proving it to be successful. I may consider some of these facts too farfetched, but I publish them as helping us to form a judgment on the experiment, and leave it to my readers to form their own. One thing I do consider to be proved by this series of experiments, and that is, that a great many of the statements of the medium could only be due to information gained supernormally.

I particularly want to draw attention to the fact that unless specially stated in the reports, all the actions and talk during the experiments were confined to the medium and myself. This excluded the possibility of suggestive questions being put to him in experiments, where the object was unknown to me and known to someone present. No signs (nods, etc.) were given.

I will begin by describing a few psychoscopic experiments with Miss von B. performed on the same evening as my last experiments with her in clairvoyance. In all these experiments the object was known to one or more of those present, unless the contrary is stated.

79th Experiment. Object. A small heart-shaped dish (Schale) which belonged to my wife. A number of these dishes had been presented to the ladies at my sister-in-law's wedding. The wedding took place on an estate in 1904 ; so I was fairly sure that she would recall a good many facts about it.

The others present knew nothing about the object. I wrapped it up in several layers of tissue paper and handed it to Miss von B. She gazed into a glass filled with water (so-called " crystal-gazing ").

It is certainly wise to refrain from passing a judgment on crystal-gazing till you have had some practical experience of it. The function of the crystal can be compared to that of the ascending main of a pumping station. It is a method which persons of a certain constitutional type use to bring certain parts of their subconscious knowledge to the surface, causing among other things supernormal phenomena. Miss von B. has had some remarkable cases of crystal vision in which she always used the crystal only as an aid to clairvoyance.[1]

"A great many flowers, baskets, bouquets, tall ones, full of flowers. Something like the hubbub of a crowd? Now it is developing. There must be a great many people. All wearing light clothes, masses of light. Masses of flowers. A lady comes to the fore wearing a light dress, fair (has a clear laugh) ; a gentleman gives her a kiss. The lady is gone.—*Trees, an alley, a garden,* no more people.—*A great many people wearing light clothes out of doors, also officers in uniform, like a party, it must be a wedding. I see a long white thing on a lady in the crowd."*

We cannot deny that this description is very good. It is possible that Miss von B. could feel the shape of

[1] The facts which could be tested or which could reasonably be considered correct from our knowledge of the history of the object are printed in italic type. I shall treat some of the facts in detail in commenting on the experiments, but only when the facts have a great degree of probability and are important. So the reader must not in any case consider the facts not specially mentioned in the commentary to be inaccurate.

the dish through the paper, but she could not conclude from this what its history was ; a heart-shaped dish could have quite a different history. The " long white thing on a lady " can I think be taken as the train or veil of the bride. There were a number of officers in uniform present at the wedding. It was not possible to find out whether the episode of the kiss was correct, but it does not seem improbable. *Positive.*

80*th Experiment.* Object : a letter balance I had received from a lady seven years ago. I handed it to Miss von B. just as it was, and made no comment.

" Like a woman's head. She is looking through an open door into a room. A woman seen from behind ; always something feminine, nothing masculine about it.—*Now I see Mr. Tischner,* he is standing opposite me, I also see a *woman's form* ; she is turning her back to me ; *she gives something to him.* Something funny, a curious *lady, profile, brunette, pale, decidedly pretty, dark dress, turned-up nose, she is holding a letter-balance in her hand. Her hair is rich and full. The lady* does not strike you as very refined, *rather common,* hair elaborately made up, more like a shop-girl, *not very ladylike,* now she has gone.—Again a lady, looks as if she belonged to a better class than the previous one, the same as the first. She is sitting in the same room, writing. There is a table with a thick green cloth on it. She has very loose hair, and is nicer than the previous one.''

The lady who gave me the balance was a decided brunette, pale, with a turned-up nose, and a mass of beautiful hair ; her dress was generally plain and dark. She would quite naturally answer the description of the second lady who held the balance in her hand. On the other hand, I know of nobody who could have been the original of the first and third ladies described in connexion with the balance. The result is striking, even if much is said which it is impossible to check or which seems to be wrong ; this is usually the case in this class of experiments. I might have come by an ordinary brass letter-balance with a curved scale in quite a different way ; and yet the description of the second lady fits the giver very well. *Positive*.

We now come to a series of psychoscopical experiments with another medium, Mr. H., a gentleman of 42 with a university education. Mr. H. has a strong psychopathological tendency and shows clear symptoms of dissociation of personality. I am told that he has had spontaneous cases of pure clairvoyance and foresight of the future ; but I shall not mention these as they do not interest us now. He has a twofold attitude towards the phenomena he produces : he regards them in a critical way, but cannot quite help being influenced by the fact that he apparently receives messages from several different personalities, containing facts which he says he could not have foreseen, and has no further knowledge of, but which prove to be correct in the majority of cases. He often uses the spiritistic mode of expression ; we cannot say much against it as it is often very convenient. The sceptic will probably say that a definite theory or mode of interpreting the facts should not be allowed to play a part in an experimental investigation, especially at so early a stage. It is apt to destroy the requisite frame of mind. I have never allowed these utterances and opinions of the medium to influence me or my experiments in the very least. I have known H. for nearly two years, both in friendly intercourse and in the séance room, and have never had any cause to doubt his sincerity and perfect honesty ; but even if he had felt the wish to deceive us I do not believe he would have succeeded, as he is so childish and clumsy. All the people who took part in the experiments share my opinion on both these points. The sceptic will say that these amiable and apparently friendly people are often the most dangerous. But the experiments, especially the later ones, were conducted in a way which made fraud impossible (see p. 110) ; I wish to repeat that he never had access to any parcel except the one he held during the experiment, and that he was not left alone with them even for a second.

H. always suffered from changeable moods and often felt very poorly. He had a slight stroke in February, 1920 ; he was not in Munich at the time. This prevented sittings for a long while. When, after a few months, we were able to take up our experiments again, he still felt ill, now and then had fits of hysterical laughter and periods of stupor of varying length ; subsequently his condition became much worse so that we had to put an end to our experiments. Now he has all the symptoms of *paralysis agitans*, which is probably due to an affection of the *globus pallidus*. The later experiments were carried out under very trying conditions ; this makes the results obtained all the more startling. H. liked the experiments, although he needed a great deal of persuasion to come to them, suffering as he did from powerful inhibitions which led him to put them off frequently for all sorts of trivial reasons. When the experiments were successful, it flattered his pride and made him feel better. He might come looking worn, and wake up as the evening went on till he was fresh and lively towards the close of the sitting. He often said the sittings did him good, maintaining that my "Od[1]" helped him. He was very willing to try the single experiments, but later on he was often in such a state of stupor that he had to be roused from it ; this had to be done, but on the other hand, it tended to spoil the results, as these sub-conscious outflows should be allowed to come quite naturally and not be urged on. H.'s inhibitions often prevented him saying all that came to him in the later

[1] Magnetic emanation (Reichenbach).

experiments ; I shall draw attention to this several times.

It is interesting to note that H. often did not know who had packed the object, i.e. the persons who knew the contents of the parcel ; and, in a number of cases, he was not personally acquainted with them. Both these conditions were fulfilled in the first " unknown " experiments where Gruber and Hattingberg were present. He made the acquaintance of Mrs. Gruber later on. The above conditions were both again fulfilled in experiments 155 and 161. I mention this here as it may be of use when we consider the paramnestic theory.

These facts seem to me to speak against the theory which assumes that nearly all the phenomena of clairvoyance are due to telepathy. I think that we can put down the above cases of psychoscopy to clairvoyance, even if they do not actually prove the absence of telepathy, in the sense in which it is used by the theory of an all-pervading telepathic faculty. If it be thought that the medium can get into touch with the person who wrote a slip, even if it were picked from several, so that no one present knows which it was, then I have not proved the absence of telepathy. It would, however, be easy to make experiments which would clear up this point, and I hope to carry them out as soon as I get a chance. But this all-embracing theory of telepathy seems to me so wide, so complicated, so fantastic, that we might expect its exponents to bring the proof of its validity, considering it is yet quite unproven.

I had held sittings for physical phenomena several times, without any results, except raps, beyond criticism. Once when we were not able to hold a sitting for physical phenomena, as we had arranged, owing to outside circumstances, I asked H. to try psychoscopy, which was quite new to him.

H. asked me to make hypnotic passes or to give

him suggestions several times; occasionally I did so on my own initiative. In both cases he does not fall into a regular hypnotic trance, but brings himself into an auto-hypnotic condition with the help of my passes and suggestions. Both these auto-hypnotic states and his trances vary in depth, and often he comes out of them quite suddenly without any external aid ; they are followed by amnesia. It is very rare that he has any recollection of what took place in these states ; these recollections are auditive. He remembers the very highly pitched voice or the very low tones of his trance utterances. This series of experiments with Mr. H. has one particular point of interest ; he had never done any experiments of this kind before those here reported, and did none with anybody else during this whole series ; this allows us to follow the evolution of this faculty of his from beginning to end.

81st *Experiment.* Present : Mrs. R., Miss O., Mr. N., H., and myself. Object : a small watch-glass with a burning heart and Mr. R.'s Christian name etched on it with hydrofluoric acid during a practical course in chemistry. Mr. R. was then engaged to Mrs. R. They were divorced when the experiment took place.

I had asked Mrs. R. for some suitable object for the experiment, and she had handed this to me. I wrapped it up in thick notepaper so that its shape could only be felt roughly.

" *A woman's head, fair, a sensation of heat, a white dress with a buckle or belt—a tennis-court*—a sensation as if there were something painted—two gloves, dull yellow, glacé, a gem with a finely cut woman's head on it. *Summer resort, health resort* —sunshine —straw hats, blue sky—*Something is past—a gentleman fair, with a pointed face*—this hand gave it to the lady and she wears it. A gentleman and a lady, but the gentleman does not care for the lady, he is ardent, but domineering, not at one with himself—large book with lots of figures, he is counting money—*disunion*—the lady is annoyed by this perpetual counting of figures, by this matter-of-fact business-like manner, she blames him—a hearse connected with the gentleman."

As far as I know we can take the following statements as correct : Mrs. R. is fair, the sensation of heat might be ascribed to the feelings of an engaged couple. The white dress with a belt might be interpreted in two ways ; this shows how misleading interpretations can be : it might apply to the gentleman's laboratory coat (long white or drab, as surgeon's coats are generally worn for chemical work in Germany) or to the lady's tennis skirt. It was not possible to clear up this point as H. had no visual knowledge of the garment ; he said he had been told the above. The words " something is past " and " disunion " could be taken as applying to the divorce. I must add that Mr. and Mrs. R. had lived in a garden suburb, a kind of summer resort for the last few years, and that Mr. R. had fair hair and a pointed face. I cannot tell how much of the remainder is characteristic, as Mr. and Mrs. R. differed on the point. I asked both of them. In such a case, an outsider should refrain from giving an opinion.

Sceptics will find the positive yield of this experiment very meagre, the interpretations doubtful and fantastic. They are not altogether wrong ; especially as a good deal could have been concluded by guesswork. Mr. H. did not know that Mrs. R. was divorced, but he might have concluded that she was either divorced or a widow, as Mrs. R. came to sittings without her husband, and it would be strange for him not to be visible in her flat; in which case he might have expected an object connected with Mr. R.[1] So we will not stress the result of this experiment. *Positive.*

---

[1] He heard later on that Mr. R. was divorced. See Experiment 109. [*Trans.*]

82nd Experiment. Object : a small oval looking-glass about 4 in. by $1\frac{1}{2}$ in., wrapped up in strong paper. I asked Mr. N. for something two rooms from the one in which H. was sitting. He handed me the above, saying that it had been given to him by a young widow whom he had met at a watering place where he stayed as a soldier. She had given it to him as a memento when he left. I wrapped it up in strong paper, took it into the room, and handed it to H.

" *A looking-glass, a woman's hand*—a picture in the looking-glass, a small oval pastel—something grey— *a girl's face, brunette, a field-grey uniform, the lady is young, under thirty—a warm shake of the hand,—a parting*—a bouquet to the gentleman—a painted photo—*a parting gift before a journey—parting, sadness. It is something that you are very fond of, have often held in your hand, there is much love connected with it, when taken up in times of trouble it brings a feeling of comfort. Worn for years* alone in a dug-out, *interlaced hands,* love by relationship or *earthly love. The face suddenly grows old, motherly, a mother. Protection and love. Something good and loving about it, something soothing that does good.*"

Although I kept on encouraging H. to say all he saw, he had refrained from doing so in both this and the previous experiment, as he lacked self-confidence and found it useless to describe all these vague visions which he thought could have no connexion with the object.

Mr. N., who had expressed his surprise during the course of the experiment by exclamations such as " capital ", etc., without giving any actual indications, now volunteered the following information : The lady was 28, brunette ; the range and intensity of their feelings had been described with great accuracy ; the glass had been given to him with the wish that he should think of the donor whenever he looked into it ;

he had not been at the Front since he left her. The lady died one year later ; on her death-bed she aked her mother to give him a farewell message. This might explain the sudden disappearance of the young face and the appearance of a motherly face. *Positive.*

NEXT SITTING

83rd Experiment. I used a chance visit to H.'s to try an experiment.

Object : a button off a ship's doctor's uniform, worn by my father on a journey to America about 50 years ago, wrapped up in paper.

" Does not belong to you—a hand, but it is not on the hand—a slender hand—a tall dark man—a large store—things under glass cases—a gentleman and a lady—the lady has auburn hair—full figure—a brush."

Tischner : " It is not a jewel as you seem to think." H. asks me to make a few magnetic passes, as I had done in previous sittings. As I made the second pass he said :

" *I keep on seeing water—as if something was being fished out—the sea. Fishermen—all is blurred—nets, the inside of the sea—sea animals—a Southern land— palms—deep blue sky—fire, clouds of dark smoke— men with hands covered with soot—now I see nothing more.*"

This can be taken as a fair description of the surroundings and happenings on a liner between Hamburg and New York. He said that he had not actually seen fire, but had concluded that it must be there from the smoke. *Positive.*

NEXT SITTING

84th–86th Experiments. Negative.

The whole of this sitting was negative ; not a single statement made which could be checked was found correct or could be considered as probably correct. H. said he was badly disposed at the very start. We

81

gave him three things and then brought the sitting to an end. I think there is no object in publishing the reports of these three experiments.

87th Experiment. Object : a paper parcel containing a small Japanese hammered and chased metal match-box. It had been given to me fifteen years ago by a duchess, a Japanese by birth.

I expected H. to describe scenes in Japan or from the life of the donor, but the experiment proved completely negative. I will give it here as an example of a negative experiment. H. was in a light hypnotic trance.

" Temple hall with white columns, people with long robes—Romans, Egyptians with long beards. Women half naked, stripped to the waist. Slabs of mosaic, then you go down as if you wanted to go down into the water. A hall with Gothic arches. Monastery or heathen temple. Brilliantly coloured. Modern people —a tall thin gentleman, a graceful lady with a grey veil and a mackintosh, a Roman face, a pretty nose, long wavy dark hair tied into a knot at the back."

At most, the " people with long robes " and the " heathen temple " might be correct. *Negative.*

88th Experiment. (" Unknown ", i.e. the contents of the parcel were not known to anyone present.)

Object : a small well-gummed packet, 4 in. by 1 in. by ¾ in. which seemed to contain a cardboard box. The contents were not known.

After a few minutes' pause H. said that he could say nothing about the contents. *Negative.*

89th Experiment. Object : a rosary blessed by the Pope. I had put it into a small box to prevent H. from feeling its shape.

" A lady in pink, she has a necklace round her neck, a necklace, pearls, flashing *there is something like a star or a cross on it*—now it is beginning to look like a cross

—a white sheen like diamonds. The lady wears a very low dress, and has very beautiful shoulders. *Not a very young lady, in the thirties, a mature woman.* She is in a room with a large company. The lady is sitting on a dull yellow sofa in a room with a wall-paper with green stripes. She has auburn hair and *a very haughty expression.* She sits and waits ; there are only gentlemen in the antechamber."

What strikes us most in this case are the data about the necklace, the form of which was perfectly recognized although the material and purpose was misinterpreted. In this case the object itself would have been perceived first and not, as was usual in the psychoscopic experiments with H., the fate and surroundings. I had been given the rosary by a lady of the age indicated. The lady is rather haughty ; she conceded this indirectly by remarking : " People say I am rather haughty," when I read the record of the experiment to her. The data about the surroundings throw an interesting light on the part played by association in these experiments. The object had been recognized as a necklace with a cross ; so it was taken to be a necklace, and suitable surroundings were associated with it. This seems to speak against a possible explanation by telepathy. If I had succeeded in transmitting the object so well in this case I do not see why I should have failed so completely in transmitting its use, etc. But if we are dealing with a case of true clairvoyance, it is quite comprehensible that a medium does not give us data obtained by psychoscopy when he is, as it were, attuned for cryptoscopy, but comes to the same conclusions by association. *Positive.*

NEXT SITTING

90th Experiment. Negative.
91st Experiment. Negative.
92nd Experiment. (Unknown.) Object : the same

parcel as in Experiment No. 88 ; a tie-pin with a pearl and two diamonds.

" A railway train. An observatory, but the observatory is open, so that you can see the stars in the sky. *An old gentleman is sitting in front of the telescope. A very thin young man in a Chinese silk suit,* and a middle-sized lady in a striped summer-dress with a broad leather belt—a promenade—*a watering-place*—a great many clipped trees, the scenery has a southern character. *Water—like the sea, the Baltic—a 'cello.* The young couple in the flat of the old gentleman who was in the observatory. *The object belongs to the old gentleman,* it is there on the table. ·I see a snuff-box and a large marble pen-tray. *The object is a present from the old gentleman* to his son, *the young man.*"

I must add the following remark taken from details received later on from Mr. K. : No information could be obtained about the observatory. The object, a tie-pin with a pearl and two diamonds, is a present from an old gentleman to a young man, but the relation is not one of father and son. The pin was given Mr. K. by his great-uncle. Mr. K. is very thin, he was wearing a Chinese silk suit and was staying at Zoppot, a seaside resort on the Baltic, when he wore the pin last.

The statements about the lady could not be verified. Mr. K.'s great-uncle had a friend a 'cellist who gave musical evenings at his house once a week ; Mr. K. attended them often. His great-uncle's house was furnished luxuriously, and there were several marble bowls, but Mr. K. can remember no pen-tray to fit the description. Mr. K. thinks that the mention of the observatory in which the stars are visible through the opening in the roof, might be taken as a symbolic reference to the pearl and the diamonds, such as we find in poetry ; we cannot reject this interpretation lightly, as symbolical visions of this kind are not uncommon in dreams, and several other features of psychoscopy remind us of dreams (e.g. the mixing up of events which are separate both in space and in time). *Positive*.

NEXT SITTING

Professor Otto Baensch, who lately held the chair of philosophy at the University of Strassburg, was present ; he had brought several small things with him. He kept the record.

93*rd Experiment. Negative.*

94*th Experiment. Negative.*

H. had very clear visions, but emphasized that they had nothing to do with the object under consideration.

95*th Experiment.* Object : a small antique Greek vase belonging to my wife. I had just put it into a small cardboard box, which H. did not open during the experiment.

" The cardboard box was made in a large paper-mill in Magdeburg. The object takes us to India—Benares, the Ganges, to the water-side—the object is certainly connected with Buddha. It is awful how I keep mixing up Benares and Ganges."

H. afterwards told us that the voices had kept on saying : " Ganges on the Benares," whereas he knew that the reverse was correct.

" *A town built on hills*, slight figures going down to the water, white garments, children are bathing in a river with a foreign character. *The clothes are not European*. Sun, sun, lots of sun, seems to be *Rome* or *Naples*, *shawls*, *loose garments*, brilliant red, bare feet and legs. Soft sea sand, small row-boats, the sound of the *piffero*, the flute, a mountain melody. I am ashamed of myself. A tall figure, modern personality, comes into the room, black frock-coat, white kid gloves, sensitive lips, seems to be here on some research work, does not fit into the scene. Suddenly, a change of

TELEPATHY AND CLAIRVOYANCE

time. The people changed, the place remained. *A modern liner. The route Genoa–Naples, a cruise in the Mediterranean.* The word Amalfi comes up. The object is not of any great value, it was carried in the inside coat pocket. *On the cruise there was a very gay company on the upper deck.* Two ladies and five gentlemen, one of the ladies married to one of the gentlemen. *A cheery company belonging to intellectual circles, artists, scientists.* An old gentleman. *The object of the journey was not in any way material or mundane. The Gulf of Messina, South Italy.* Benares. It certainly is not India."

H. is very excited. Tischner calms him down and tells him that the results are satisfactory to encourage him.

" The tempter keeps on calling out Benares by which the Ganges is meant. There is a musician on board with a sketch-book in his pocket containing motives, or a text, a libretto. *A love affair, it is being spun out with great ardour between the young lady and a gentleman. A strong erotic wave. The gentleman has a big moustache and some beard on his chin, they are leaning against the rail.*"

My wife bought this vase in Athens when she was a girl. I should not like to say whether the vase is really old or not : H.'s statements about the non-European clothing might be taken as evidence of its antiquity. The route followed was really Genoa–Naples, i.e. the sea journey began in Genoa, led to the East through the Gulf of Messina, and ended up in Naples, then Rome was visited. The company was often very merry, and there really were very intimate relations between the young lady mentioned and a gentleman with a big moustache and a pointed beard ; their intimacy seems to have been somewhat overrated by H. *Positive.*

96*th Experiment.* Object : a small Turkish silver coin, packed up in tissue-paper so that you could not

86

feel what it was. Professor B. used to carry it about in his purse with two French fifty-centime pieces, a few German stamps, a box-key, and a ribbon of the Iron Cross. The coin was given to him during the war by a middle-aged lady whose brother was reported missing. She was very fond of him.

"A letter, large envelope, large thick paper. *A field-grey uniform* flashes up. They tell me, *She sat with eyes reddened by tears.*"

Interruption.

"Again I saw : (1) *A person with an Iron Cross in field-grey.*

(2) "*A death, funeral decorations, laurels.*

(3) "*Eyes red from crying*—the object was sent in a letter. Without a doubt from a foreign country. Something that was made during the war, connected with the war. ' Speak Chinese !—Speak Chinese ! ' says the evil spirit—*The object does date from earlier on, but changed hands during the war, became more precious.* Say : ' *It is a ribbon of the Iron Cross* ' ; cries the evil spirit. But this is nonsense.—*The Wars of Independence,* 1813. *A frail middle-aged woman, a very pretty thin hand.* Made of black stone, a bracelet. A small box on the table."

Baensch finds the following points in the history of the object strikingly in accord with the visions [1]:

(1) I met the lady during the war ; I was wearing a field-grey uniform at the time, and had the Iron Cross 2nd class.

(2) The lady is frail, middle-aged, and has beautiful thin hands.

---

[1] I have published B.'s commentary without any alterations, and have kept the numerical classifications of the points of agreement and divergence. I have nothing to say against the numerical classification in itself, but I should like to warn readers against basing arguments on the fact that an experiment has, say, four positive and four negative statements, and so is neither positive nor negative. These factors do not compensate each other, and a really characteristic statement cannot be outweighed by ever so many negative ones.

(3) She misses her only brother very much.

(4) The object does come from a foreign country, but not from China ; the Thugra [1] on the coin reminds one strongly of Chinese writing.

(5) The coin is from 30 to 40 years old, but changed hands during the war and did change value as it has different values for the lady and for me.

(6) I carried it in my purse with a ribbon of the Iron Cross. The Iron Cross was first given in the Wars of Independence.

It is not possible to find out if the object was sent in a letter or to get any data relating to the black bracelet or the box. No connexion could be found with the funeral decorations or the laurels, as the funeral never took place. (This statement may possibly have a symbolical meaning only. See my remarks on p. 84.— Tischner.) It is not true that the object had a connexion with the war. However, this was corrected by the medium later on ; it is true of the ribbon though. So far, Professor B., I must say that I consider the experiment decidedly positive. *Positive.*

NEXT SITTING

Present : Professor Baensch, H., and myself.

97*th Experiment.* Object : a written slip which I had picked out from several without knowing which I had taken. I had wrapped it up in two layers of dark purple paper and put it into an envelope made of paper with print on the inside, and closed it with a strip of gummed paper.

It was quite impossible to recognize a single line through the envelope, even against a strong light. I told H. that it contained a few verses. H. said at once :

---

[1] The seal of the Sultan, which is on every Turkish stamp and coin.

EXPERIMENTS

" Longing wafts gently into the night from an evening sky. Evening mood, melancholia, longing for peace. Hebbel's ' Nachtlied ', Goethe, soft welling mood, a song of longing rings forth, a gentle bell. ' I send,' this is being read, ' many flowers to you '."

On opening we found four lines of Goethe's *Wand'rers Nachtlied :*

> Ach ! Ich bin des treibens müde !
> Was soll all der Schmerz und Lust ?
> Süsser Friede—
> Komm, ach komm in meiner Brust.[1]

After the experiment was over H. said very emphatically: " I find the general feeling of the poem very well rendered." *Positive.* He had said the word " Goethe " meaning that the *Nachtlied* was written by Goethe, so this was meant to correct the statement that it was Hebbel's *Nachtlied.*

Professor Becher, who holds the chair of philosophy at the University of Munich, joined us after this experiment.

98th Experiment. Object : a bottle of Eau de Cologne given to Professor Baensch by a third person. It was packed in a cardboard box.

This experiment must be considered as negative, but we will give the record of it here as it is instructive ; it shows with what detail the data of negative experiments are often given.

" A darkly papered wall with a round picture hanging on it. I have a violent headache caused by the object. It must have something to do with electricity. I saw a curious hand. A mine had something to do with it, a dirty workman, strong, sturdy. The object was welded. Fear and distress are connected with it. It

---

[1] How weary I am of wandering.
Oh whither this joy and pain ?
Peace, sweet peace, come back to me
And fill my bosom again.

has nothing to do with the professor ; it does not fit a man like him at all. A fellow calls out : ' Birthday present.' I saw a cycle at the very beginning, a bicycle. A striking figure, thin, very thin, a student or an officer in civilian clothing, the owner of the bicycle. House, No. 41 on it, a kind of country house with a small porch, a gravel alley and a fence in front of it. A lady, the mother of the young gentleman ; the latter has a flirtation with the lady's-maid. I fancy the young man had the object with him when cycling."

B. subsequently produced the following information about the object : The Eau de Cologne was used by a lady to bathe the temples of her dying father ; he had committed suicide by poison. The statement that " fear and distress are connected with it " might have been meant in this connection. It is also correct that the cycle has nothing to do with me. We can find no further connexions between what he said and the object. *Negative.*

99*th Experiment. Negative.*

I had chosen the object. The statements made were not sufficiently descriptive of the object or closely enough connected with it to lead us to call it a positive experiment.

100*th Experiment.* Object (unknown) : Baensch hands H. a small cardboard box. On opening it at the end of the experiment we found the ticket to a ball to which the lady who gave the parcel to Baensch had been.

" *A thin fair lady*, middle-aged, sitting at a sewing-table, unmarried. She has a great many books in her flat, two rooms, a double door like a library, chairs. *She does not live alone. The object belongs to the lady* and was lying on the sewing-table, with coloured silk ribbons. There is a flower-stand in her drawing-room. A particularly quiet and peaceful atmosphere. The lady is musical, plays the piano, long fingers, a ring with a sapphire on her finger, has bad eyesight, *rather lifeless eyes*, not so pretty as she is *kind, serious, thick-blooded.*"

Baensch says that the following particulars are correct :

(1) The lady is thin, fair, only 22, but looks ten years older, not married.

(2) She was engaged in the book trade, and has a small, very choice, library of her own.

(3) She lives with a friend.

(4) The object belongs to the lady.

(5) The lady is quiet, kind, serious and thick-blooded.

(6) She wears a ring.

The following statements have no connexion with the lady, or are not correct :

(1) She does not possess a sewing-table, and has not sat at one for a long time.

(2) The description of the flat does not apply to any of the flats she has lived in during the last few years.

(3) The lady is not particularly musical ; she does not play any instrument ; her fingers are not particularly long.

(4) The stone in her ring is a chrysoprase, not a sapphire.

(5) Her sight is very good, although her eyes are rather lifeless.

I am also of the opinion that more has been seen than could be attributed to chance ; the lady's character was described very correctly. The statement that she has a great many books can probably be regarded as positive ; it may have been a symbolical mode of expression, as in dreams, showing her connexion with the book-trade, or she may actually have been seen in the book-shop. *Positive ?*

101*st Experiment. Negative.*

102*nd Experiment.* Object (unknown) : Baensch hands a box to H. He does not know its contents. B. ascertained on inquiry that the contents were a ring made from a copper shell-ring at the front. A heart was engraved on it. It belonged to the lady who gave us the bottle mentioned in the previous experiment, but was given by the lady mentioned in Experiment No. 100.

" Again the same personality as in the last experiment but one (No. 100). Object : a brooch, given her by a gentleman. I keep hearing them call ' Lolo '. *A small locket* on a black velvet ribbon, *the locket seems to contain a photo.* There is another tugging at me again. The lady causes herself pain. I see with distress a finely-strung soul not finding her fulfilment in a man. ' Alas ! Two souls dwell in my breast.' *The object brings back reminiscences to the lady.* A vain call for happiness. I am made to suffer in sympathy with this object."

H. puts down the packet. We open it and find a ring in it. H. adds :

" The ring comes from a person who was dear to her. The ring certainly did hang round her neck on a black velvet ribbon."

B. made the following comments on the object. Accurate statements :

(1) It was given to the lady by a gentleman.

(2) The lady was given a locket with a photo by this gentleman.

(3) She did care very much for this gentleman. He was killed in the war.

Inaccurate statements :

(1) The lady is not fair like the lady of Experiment No. 100, she has black hair, and is a Jewess.

(2) The object is not a brooch.

(3) " Lolo " is unknown to both ladies.

(4) The locket is on a gold chain, but it is never worn by the lady.

(5) The ring has never been worn on a velvet ribbon.

(6) Neither of these ladies shows a degree of suffering

above or below that which is normal under their circumstances. Perhaps we can call the experiment weakly positive. *Half Positive.*

NEXT SITTING

Present : Professor Baensch, Professor E. von Aster, Professor of Philosophy, Dr. Flaskämper, and myself. H. told me at once that he had tried to ring me up to put off the sitting as the illness of his child and professional worries had made his frame of mind unfit for experiments ; but he had not been able to get the connexion. As a matter of fact my telephone was out of order. As all were present, we decided to try a few experiments.

103rd–105th Experiments. Negative.

H. gave us much detailed information, which however did not seem to apply to the objects in hand, so we will only consider No. 106, the last experiment that evening. as some of it might be taken as positive if judged with great leniency.

106th Experiment. Object (unknown) : An envelope containing a note, written by me ; it had been picked out of a good many by Professor v. Aster.

" Only tomfoolery—desire and love are the fetishes leading to greater deeds—bubbling mirth, champagne, student life."

On opening we found Heine's verses :

Am Tische war noch ein Plätzchen
Mein Liebchen da hast Du gefehlt
Du hättest so hübsch, mein Schätzchen
Von Deiner Liebe erzählt.[1]

Positive.

Incidentally, I should like to mention that it is very striking that the results should have been so bad on

[1] There was still one place at the table
My darling I missed thee there.
My sweet ! Oh just to be able
To hear of thy love so fair.

93

a day when Mr. H. was not feeling up to the mark and wanted to put off the séance. If all this were no more than pure coincidence, and H.'s statements only depended on chance, then I do not see why the results of this séance should be worse than those of any other. The objection that these results depend on guesswork, and that this faculty failed on that particular day does not hold good. Mr. H. must have realized that the objects generally came from persons he did not know, and they were all well packed up, so that guesswork could hardly play any part at all. On the other hand, if we assume that he depends on some special gift or power for his information, it would seem quite natural for this faculty to be absent, as he felt it probably would be, and that the answers should be mainly due to chance, which actually was the case.

Next Sitting

This was held at H.'s. Professor Baensch, Mr. R., Doctor of Philosophy, H., and I were present. Dr. R. took down the record in shorthand.

I handed R. several written slips, some purple paper, and an envelope. He turned his back to H., pulled a slip out of the bundle, wrapped it up in purple paper, and put it in the envelope without looking at it.

107th Experiment. Object : a slip with Hebbel's poem :

Dies ist ein Herbsttag, wie ich keinen sah !
Die Luft ist still, als atmete man kaum
Und dennoch fallen raschelnd, fern und nah
Die schönsten Früchte ab von jedem Baum.[1]

H. said at once : " Golden autumn stubble field, stubble-field of death, autumn."

[1] An autumn day as ne'er I'd seen.
As without breath the air so still
Yet crashing, rustling on the green,
Its finest fruits each tree doth spill.

94

EXPERIMENTS

He wanted to give up the experiment, so we opened the envelope. *Positive.*

108*th Experiment.* Object (unknown) : One of the above slips.

The description given did not tally with the contents of the slip. *Negative.*

H. either felt the contents of these slips at once, or did not get any data right at all.

109*th Experiment.* (Object known to Dr. R.) Object : the wedding ring of Dr. R. packed up in a small box 3 in. by 3 in. by ¾ in., wrapped in white paper and tied up with string. It was handed to H. by Dr. R.

" A field, a beautiful field with flowers, the end of spring. May, June, I see butterflies most markedly. A couple are walking across the field—*a fair lady*, in a sky blue dress—I see a *thin gentleman* with her. I see it so clearly that I am led to conclude that the scene takes place in Thuringia, I should almost like to say Eisenach ; ' The sun is high ' is called out to me. I suddenly see the lady in a room with modern furniture, standing at a window, reading a letter. She puts something into her dress here (showing his breast), and elderly lady comes through the folding door, grey hair, wears a white cloth with lace on her bodice, fichu with lace, ruche with lace, I see a table with a plush cloth on it, a lace centre runs down the middle of it, with a long streak in the middle of it, there is a marble or glass bowl on it, in which you can put fruit, but there is no fruit in it. I don't know whether these are visiting cards. *Much affection must have been attached to this object, it was kept with much reverence, there is love connected with it.* It must have been worn here (pointing to his breast). It seems to me to be a letter, a written memento, because it was hidden here (the breast). They call to me that the lady gives it back to the gentleman, either the one she received it from or another one ; that not unwillingly pressed by an urgent desire—*I have the impression that the heart of the lady is bound to it*, but she gives it back, she parts from it—*there is so much warmth connected with it*—did she do it under the influence of the elderly lady ? It happened in her room. I like the window, a quiet, peaceful corner. Now suddenly I see a well-lit concert-hall, this is not possible is it ? Just before I had the impression that the lady held the ring in her hand."

We then stopped the experiment. After a short pause we tried another experiment which is described below, then we went on with this one. H. gave us a few impressions he had had before taking the object into his hand :

He had begun by seeing live butterflies, *then he saw large exotic butterflies in a collection, also smaller ones not exotic, Death-heads, Swallow-tails, there was a particularly beautiful blue one, sky blue, exotic, in the middle, then smaller yellow ones with black markings.*

He took the object in his hand.

" The same room again, two windows facing towards the street, a small patch of garden, a quiet street, nice and shady, a good deal of curtain, green cloth, gobelin —small tables between the windows, small curios, porcelains, a vase ; lower down, animals ; fine porcelain, a door leads out of the room, there seems to be another room next to it, which seems to belong to a dentist, no, like a laboratory, but not a doctor's."

H. stands up and walks about as if he thinks he is in a room, and wants to have a thorough look at it.

" I see *books, various kinds of tubes, glasses and small apparatus, glass outer tubes, outer tubes of aluminium, I see a balance, a book-shelf along the back wall, with books on it*, not literature, mathematical signs—*Title, Chemistry, Text-book*, they call out ' Bunsen ' to me— now I am biased. I see another interesting book, it has something to do with *physics*, a number of publications all alike—Roman type, the whole library, 10, 12, 14, 15, it stops here, what a pity. No, there is more, a large number of publications, about one of the exact sciences, but it is not in German, it is in English, American, technical, good Lord! how silly! A regular laboratory."

H. goes back to his seat and comes out of trance ; he does not know that he has been walking about. Pause.

"Now I see the two together again, *they kiss each other, still a young man and a fair-haired creature, a girl.* Yes, they might be married, or he is a boarder in their house, or mother and daughter. *But they are in love with one another*, in any case—Oh! *she gives him a ring*, the thing she keeps hidden away there (see above) *is a ring. There is something engraved on it, but oddly enough on the inside*—I, G,—I think I even see *a date* on it—all very small—not a common ring—but all this happens in the room."

R. : "Do you see anything more on the ring?"

"It is as if there were a relief on it, strange scratches, thicker in the middle than at the sides, but there is no stone on it, more like a signet-ring or like a ring with a coat of arms. *The lady parted with the ring and gave it to the gentleman*, but the ring itself did not like it— *the lady parted with the ring, not against her will, but forced to do it by the circumstances—she herself was attached to the ring*—the ring is torn in two inwardly. I see a conveyance with boxes ; they call to me : ' he *is moving, she is moving '—it came to a quarrel* and one of them is leaving the house and calling out to me : ' *He is going, he is leaving the house*,'—The other is calling to me : ' *She is leaving*, he has shown her the door.' *Separation, separation, separation*—either they are married, or she lives with her mother, and he was their boarder, I rather think they might be married, but I don't understand why the elderly lady is there—perhaps the elderly lady is the owner or landlady of the boarding-house—I only see a servant, white apron, a little fat thing—there is a nice couch in the room, a sort of rocking-chair, oddly enough, I am sitting on it."

H. rocks on his chair.

" In a green room—the ladies' room—the furniture is slightly greenish, modern, small rocking chair, next this another room, a dining-room with carved furniture, coloured light, there is a light rug under the dinner-table, greyish ; the furniture is light, and made of oak."

Dr. R. made the following remarks : " It is quite astonishing how many of these statements can be brought into connexion with the object and with the lives of my divorced wife and myself. The scene first described with the fair-haired (correct) young lady, and the thin (correct) young man on a field towards the end of spring, could be taken as a description of our first meeting. This was between Schliersee and Tegernsee on a botanical excursion which took place on 17th May. (Mrs. R. was then studying medicine.) The supposition that the scene took place in Thuringia is erroneous, unless another incident impressed itself upon H.'s mind ; our stay at my mother's in Nieder-Lösznitz near Dresden a year later, in April or May ; or is the first picture connected with this stay ? The butterflies in the collection would seem to point to that, the description fits the collection I had at home as a child. (It is strange in what an inconsequent way this description follows on to what preceded it.) The elderly lady with grey hair may be taken for my mother, the white fichu with lace would be correct, so would the description of the table with the velvet cloth and the bowl. But I don't wish to overrate the importance of this first part. (The butterfly collection excepted.) It is obvious that the italicized words from ' A great deal of affection ' to ' there is love connected with it ' fit the object perfectly. The impression that the object is a letter or something similar is corrected subsequently by the fact that the ring is seen. The remarks beginning with ' The lady gives ' to ' so much warmth connected with it ' are a very good allusion to the part played by it. The description of the laboratory is important ; the italicized data fit truly the scientific laboratory I had furnished in the room next to my study in the first flat we lived in after getting married. The foreign publications seen by H. are a mistake. The next italicized statements are obviously correct. A date and some letters are actually engraved on it, there is no ' G ' but two ' i's '. That my asking H. whether he saw any more details of the ring should have caused him to make a few erroneous statements may be due to my question having a suggestive effect on his imagination, as he may have thought that there was more to be seen (it was a normal wedding-ring of uniform width). H.'s words from ' He is moving ' to ' quarrel ' then ' separation ' can be taken as describing the divorce. ' He has shown her the door ' might symbolize that I definitely suggested the divorce (the actual statement was not correct !)."

I should like to add a few remarks to Dr. R.'s commentary. H. knew that R. was divorced, so as soon as he knew that it was a ring, he could have made a good many of his statements without any further visions. The strange thing is that a faculty allowed him to be led in the right direction to state "it is a ring" by the packet, a thing none of us could guess, and then to make correct statements about its fate. H. only knew that R. was a philosopher, and did not know that he had been a scientist earlier on, so the description of the laboratory is most surprising. The apparently contradictory statements " he is moving ", " she is moving ' might convey the idea that although R. was the one to take the first steps for the divorce, Mrs. R.

first suggested it, as she herself told me. So we can take the descriptions of the butterfly collection, the laboratory, then the discovery of the ring, and of the different frames of mind which led to the divorce, as being the most remarkable features of the experiment. *Positive.*

110th *Experiment.* Object : the rosary of experiment No. 89, packed up in a spectacle case.

The experiment took place in a pause of the previous experiment. H. said immediately :

" I think I am worried by the spectacle case. I see the Pope. They call to me, ' You must say " I see the Pope ".' I saw a brilliant white form."

As the most important things about the object had been said, I decided to break off the experiment. It was to be expected that he would be so influenced by this that he would see scenes to fit this. The object had been given to him in the same case last time, so that an association of ideas is not quite impossible. However, this seems very improbable, as this very spectacle case had been used for several other experiments without his seeing the Pope. We used the same packings for different objects several times without detecting any disturbing influence at all. This experiment falls into line with other ones, so we can consider it as strikingly positive. *Positive.*

NEXT SITTING

Present : Professor Baensch, Dr. R., Mrs. T., Mrs. H., H., and I.

111th *Experiment.* Object (unknown) : an envelope containing a few verses. *Negative.*

112th *Experiment.* (Known to Dr. R.) Object : Mrs. R.'s wedding-ring ; it had been put into a cardboard box $2\frac{1}{2}$ in. by $2\frac{1}{2}$ in. by $\frac{1}{4}$ in., which was then wrapped up in blue paper. I handed it to H.

EXPERIMENTS

H. had visions of a party. These were interrupted at intervals by a new personality who calls himself " Skutter ". He appeared for the first time at this sitting, and speaks English with a very good accent. When he speaks German he has a strong English accent, and often puts English words into his conversation. A pause—then H. says :

" A very fine old chest of drawers—old fittings, very fine metal work, a visiting-card with *Elfriede*—now I see a lady and an elderly gentleman, father and daughter—this is the impression I have—*the lady is fair*—the elderly gentleman has rather a rosy face, side whiskers, pepper and salt, turning grey a humorous face, and wears glasses—the lady is difficult to describe, fair, middle-sized."

H. says with a broad Bavarian accent and quite a different voice. H. is not a Bavarian :

" ' larded ', as the Bavarian would say, full about the hips."

Tischner : " Where do you see the two ? "

" Switzerland—Switzerland. Now it has all melted away. Now I see a jewel case."

Tischner : " What does it look like ? "

" The lady wears a ' Reformkleid '.[1] I cannot distinguish her features—*a strong erotic wave comes from this object.* The lady has a pendant on her watch chain, *a tiny notebook*, I think that she has either just taken it out of the case or put it in. *This little silver thing has ivory pages, little slates.* The picture remains the same. *There is no sense of joy attached to the object—* I mean the thing in the packet. *An impression of discontent given by the lady in her room.* ' *Pensive—elle est très pensive—il est très merveilleux de voir les*

---

[1] The " Reformkleid " or reform dress is a loose garment, without a waist, but two braces over the shoulders ; it is not as long as a robe, and was introduced into Central Europe as a reaction to tight lacing about twenty years ago.

secrets les plus profondes de l'âme humaine. *It seems to me a very bitter-sweet memory.*' Why all these calls to-day, why is it not me to-day? "

H. had the impression that most of these things were being said to him.

" Très pensive—she is brooding—*struggling to gain her independence—two beings, two worlds, two worlds in her innermost—they are quarrelling with one another—* it interests me very much—*a very warm erotic wave goes out from her,* a wave which she does not herself understand. A very beautiful lady—I am Skutter— nothing more, a foreign town. It is so awkward to say it, the Englishman is speaking to you madam."

To Mrs. Tischner : . . . Pause. H. is dissatisfied ; R. wants to encourage him, and tells him that although the result was negative to begin with, many of the statements made later do fit the object. Now H. knows that the object comes from R.

" I can't get on, I see the lady again sitting at a table with a jewel-case, *and it is a ring,* she either puts it into the case or puts it on, and *is brooding, pensive—* the Frenchman is chatting with the Englishman— *decidedly a ring.*"

H. said this in a sceptical tone. Tischner says : " The statement may be correct " to encourage him.

" A new picture—the lady is sitting writing a letter. 'Damned Germany—I detest you—I detest Germans—',"turning to Mrs. T. (this was said in English).

" ' Always to first the ladies ' (in English) . . . She has a *quite masculine library.*"

T. : " Please, how do you mean masculine ? "

" *Scientific books.* I see *literature, medicine, natural science.*"

T. : " In a book-case ? "

" No, partly on the writing-table, at which she is writing."

T. : " Can you describe the room ? "

EXPERIMENTS

" Very light furniture, the table almost white, yellowish—*something in alcohol*, I can't quite see what it is, part of a tape-worm ? "

T.: " Perhaps you can describe the lady, the room, the frame of mind the lady is in."

" Nothing at all . . . *she must be a student*—I think I see her going up the steps of the university—strangely enough it seems to me to be Würzburg, a modern building—suddenly, the same lady having a pleasant conversation in the passage of the university—a portfolio under her arm—*he is rather taller than she*, fair—now she is wearing something like a man's collar, at least I fancy a blue tie—they call to me Giordano Bruno and Walter Pater, Renaissance . . ."

Pause in which another experiment is tried (No. 113).

" Electric tram—nothing more to be done—the lady parts with the ring—she presents it to a gentleman—she makes an actual present of it—but out of love—a happy frame of mind—I don't understand what the ring is supposed to do—*she strokes the gentleman here* (*showing the back of his head*) *soothingly, gently—they* call to me : town in North Germany—*now I see a wedding, carriages stop, the two drive away, a newly-married couple—she was brooding again just now*—away from the house—out of a flat—this seems to take place in a town in North Germany—*he probably made her acquaintance at the university*—I only wish I could follow the journey—it is not a journey at all—it is only a neighbouring town—now they live together—again in a private house—*not a very large house—their landing has only three or four windows on the front of the house*—but they live together, they are married. There is no instrument in the flat—they called ' violin ' to me—but I do not accept this as I do not see a violin—it is finished . . . *Now both have sad faces—each one is by himself*—she goes away, travels back to the neighbouring town—all this is madness—(Skutter :) your wife will leave before Christmas . . . send money for meat—don't buy the expensive hare or the Landshuters will make long noses . . ." This was obviously to Mrs. H.

Skutter (in broken German) : " Thing left behind by a pretty woman who has gone (ist gegangen)—precious relic, tender souvenir—very strongly and deeply touched, *torn apart—has departed, this is what is left of the ' heart '* (this word was said in English), good, good, ' *sweet dreams* ' (sweet dreams was in English), *reminiscences of beautiful hours, which have passed, which have gone* (sind verschwunden)."

Mrs. H. : " Emerson ? " (As Emerson had reported several times.) " Not Emerson, Skutter . . . your hand " to R., who gives it to him.

" Very good " (in English) . . . " I can't get any further to-day."

I now give Dr. R.'s commentary slightly modified and completed by inserting Mrs. R.'s notes. In so far as the italicized statements are not quite clear I wish to add that Mrs. R.'s christian name is " Frieda " ; compare this with the name " Elfriede " on the visiting card ; the description of the father is quite good but not absolutely characteristic ; the ring was wrapped up in pink cotton-wool in a rectangular box with rounded edges. Mrs. R. wore " reform-dresses " at the beginning of her married life. She did have a small silver note-book with ivory or celluloid pages on her watch-chain, but she had given up wearing it when she met R. The remarks from " There is no sense of joy " to " it seems to be a bitter-sweet memory ! " obviously refer to their married life. The beginning of their married life was a very happy one ; the bitterness only began to creep in later (bitter-sweet memory). The strong desire to struggle through to personal independence (not only pecuniary) after this unhappy marriage was often expressed by Mrs. R. The statement that two worlds are wrestling with one another in her innermost, applies to her most certainly ; more so than it could be said of most people. This very pronounced disharmony was the main cause of the unhappy marriage.

It was during the pause that H. was first told that the object came from R., so from that point guesswork might have begun playing a part to a certain extent ; however, the statements made before the pause were very characteristic, and this case was one in which it was by no means easy to come to conclusions by guesswork ; then again the last object was a ring, so that you would not naturally conclude in favour of its being one again. This points strongly to the knowledge being obtained by the same means as at the beginning, i.e. clairvoyance. Mrs. R. studied medicine before getting married, as was stated previously. The things said about the scientific and medical books are correct. The description of the preparation in alcohol is very striking, as students do not generally study preparations at home. The soothing and gentle way of stroking the back of the head is characteristic of Mrs. R. The North German town might be Bonn, where the R.'s passed the first years of their married life. It is interesting to note that H. particularly mentions a flat when speaking of the wedding and never mentions a church,which is generally the chief point of interest of a wedding. A " clairvoyant " who " sees " by guesswork would probably have seen a church. As a matter of fact no religious ceremony took place. Referring to H.'s saying " she was brooding again just now ", R. said that he could remember quite distinctly how the truly delightful happiness of her wedding day was troubled by sudden fits of melancholy brooding, an alternation quite characteristic of Mrs. R.

The wedding did not take place in the North German

TELEPATHY AND CLAIRVOYANCE

town Bonn, but in Munich. That they made each
other's acquaintance as students was mentioned above.
H. sees no journey. As a matter of fact their honey-
moon was not spent in travelling, they only moved to
Bonn. The flat in Bonn did have three windows on
the street front, one of which was a large bow-window.
There is no violin in the flat ; so far H. was right, but
there was a guitar, which being similar to a violin in
shape, might have caused the call " violin ". There
was also a piano. The italicized words from " Now "
to " alone " can be taken as referring to the disagree-
ments which were gradually creeping into their married
life.

On the whole we can say that the general note of the
object and its life is very well given, especially as the
ring was seen. This fact is of great importance if we
call to mind the object of the very last experiment
was a ring also, so that a ring would hardly be expected
to follow it immediately. It was against all
probabilities.

I lay particular stress on the jewel-case with pink
cotton-wool, the "reform-dress", the description of the
flat, then great stress on the preparation in alcohol,
and lastly on the little notebook as a pendant.

Normally H. speaks no English, he only knows very
few words, and his accent is very poor ; his pro-
nunciation in trance was remarkably good. He cannot
speak German with an English accent with any degree
of success in his normal condition. *Positive.*

113*th Experiment.* Object : Mrs. T. had brought
a small flexible oval box, without a lid, about 5½ in.
by 2½ in. by 1 in., wrapped up in tissue paper so that
you could feel its shape through the paper.

This experiment was carried out in the above mentioned pause in the previous experiment.

" Nothing at all, simply nothing at all—discomfort,
because it keeps on reminding me of a collar—a tall

gentleman wearing this collar who has a ' collarly '
fate (kragisch), not a tragic fate (tragisch), now I see
a dancer with a tambourine . . ."
This experiment clearly shows how the clairvoyant
is misled by being able to feel the object through the
paper. H. considered the experiment as negative
from the very beginning, as the shape of the parcel
reminded him of a collar and then of a tambourine.
Compare this with p. 135. *Negative.*

NEXT SITTING

In H.'s flat. Present H., Dr. and Mrs. Tischner.
114*th Experiment. Negative.*
115*th Experiment.* (Known to Mrs. T.) Object : a
paper star, drawn, cut out and painted by my daughter
when she was nearly seven ; there was a ribbon tied
to it, and it had hung on the Christmas tree. It was
packed in a small box which I handed to H.
" I only see a little child with charming, dainty little
hands, she is holding scissors and a pencil in her hands,
very girlish. I see fair hair, loose; 6 or 7 years old; I see
the dainty face. Butterflies and birds, but made of
paper, with pointed beaks . . . It was all done with
a pencil and scissors, a child's whim. Children's gloves,
all points to the child. It is all connected with the
child. A ribbon, a ' Kripperl ' (small wooden figures
representing child Jesus in the manger, Joseph, Mary,
and the shepherds)—children's hair. It seems to me
that the children's hair is woven into the work, isn't
it a little wreath of children's hair. It is a piece of work,
but I can get no further."
The child is well described, paper birds and butterflies did hang on the Christmas tree, and under it there
was a little manger with a small representation of the
scene in the stable of Bethlehem. H. had not seen the
object. This was the first experiment with H. in which
a child was the principal character, so one cannot

attribute the fact that he saw a child to a lucky guess. *Positive.*

As already mentioned, H. had a slight stroke in February, 1920. He never regained his former health, and all the experiments with the Commission of the Medical Society were somewhat spoilt by this. This happened when he was not in Munich, which prevented us from doing any experiments for a long time. When we did begin again he still felt very ill ; this feeling was without a doubt partly genuine, but there was probably a strong neurasthenic tinge as well.

At the end of April, 1920, I gave a lecture to the Munich Medical Association on my experiments. On the same evening a Commission was elected to go into the study of occult phenomena. H. was so extremely sensitive that it was not possible to allow the whole commission to be present at the sittings. It was found that even one single new face could have a detrimental influence on the results ; this might have been much more pronounced if many had been present. So only one member of the commission was present on most occasions. I naturally had to tell H. about the formation of this commission, as he would have been surprised at the sudden appearance of a number of new faces. I, for my part, think that it influenced H. at the first sittings, as he must have realized that these gentlemen were very anxious to witness phenomena, and that would make him feel that something was expected of him—a frame of mind which is decidedly prejudicial to the production of subconscious phenomena, as it suggests an increased action of the conscious will. As it happened, one of the members of the commission was present at by far the greater number of the experiments. This was Professor Karl Gruber ; so even if it was not possible for all the members of the commission to witness the phenomena, it was of advantage that one of its members saw a great deal and was able to form a judgment based on considerable experience. I should like to emphasize that Professor Gruber states he is quite convinced that the phenomena are genuine, and can be explained only by the supernormal faculties of Mr. H. 'This statement made by my most experienced collaborator should command attention, and might be expected to have more weight than objections from desk theorists who have no first-hand knowledge of the subject. We treat occultism as a science based on direct experience, and are not prepared to go into speculations as to the probability or possibility of explaining these phenomena on the grounds of deduced arguments or a priori opinions. (See page 180.)

As in most series of experiments, the method became more exact and the routine more uniform. This, however, does not diminish the value of the previous experiments, and I maintain that it does not alter their value and standard of accuracy at all.

Now all objects were wrapped up in paper and packed in small boxes (3 in. by $3\frac{3}{4}$ in. by $\frac{1}{2}$ in. or larger) so tightly that they would not move at all when the box was shaken. The boxes were then wrapped up in paper, and tied up with string crosswise as usual ; sometimes they were sealed. The dealings with the medium fell almost solely to me. Dr. Recknagel put a few questions to H. in one negative experiment, and Professor Gruber made a few remarks which are mentioned always in the reports. Whenever I made a remark about the object in an experiment, knowing what it was, the fact is also clearly stated. In experiments where members of the commission were present, I never knew what the object was, and so could not have given any positive help. I only asked H. to tell us everything he saw, and encouraged him. The members of the commission refrained from handing their parcels to H. so that they should never be led to realize their contents by their weight ; I always handed them to him, or he would take them up himself, whichever produced the most favourable " Od " (see Reichenbach). H. was always well watched ; the experiments were all carried out in a well-lighted room, and he was never allowed to open the parcels.

Mrs. H. was often present during the experiments. We could hardly help that owing to the smallness of their flat. She was quite passive ; she did not have a chance of influencing the experiments in any way owing to the manner in which they were conducted.

We carried on the experiments in which the object was known to none of us in the manner described below ; the members of the commission approved of it, and it enabled us to open the parcel after the experiment and tell H. whether or not it was successful. This was a help, as success encouraged and assisted him tremendously. One or more of the members of the commission gave their wives or some other reliable person a number of objects to choose from and pack ; this took place in their homes. Three or four of the things were packed, the others being locked up in a drawer so that the experimenters could not tell which had been chosen.

I did not restrict my experiments with H. to those with the commission, but made a series of experiments with objects mostly known to me and which gave good results now and again. I took my chances when they came, as I hoped to find out the part played by telepathy, its extent, and the nature of its influence. My results on this point are not very conclusive. *All the gentlemen who took part in or witnessed the experiments were unanimous that there could have been no fraud.*

In the experiments done with members of the commission, "(Object known)" means that one of the members of the commission present knew the objects ; I never knew what they were in that series of experiments. The records were kept always by one of the members of the commission present, Professor Gruber and Dr. von Hattingberg keeping theirs in shorthand.

SITTING OF 16TH MAY, 1920

Held in my flat.

First sitting with the commission. Present, Dr. Wilhelm Specht, nerve-specialist and professor at the university, H. and I.

H., who had been ill, was still far from well, and very self-conscious.

116*th Experiment. Negative.*

117*th Experiment. Negative.*

SITTING OF 4TH JUNE, 1920

Held in H.'s flat.

Present : Professor Gruber, H., and I.

118*th Experiment.* Object (unknown) : a Bavarian war medal.

" *A tortoise,* like a zoological garden, two forms appear—I keep on sensing a *tortoise,* large ones, *tortoises,* now they are being fed with green stuff.

" *A tall gentleman with a fair beard,* a lady and two children are walking in the garden—wears a yellow suit, brown shoes, and a tallish straw hat—*a kind of tropical suit*—the zoological garden is not in Germany, I feel it—they call out Amsterdam to me—there certainly is *something tropical* about it. I refuse to accept Heligoland ! Not over the seas—he seems to me to be an *explorer—he comes from a hot country.* How can he be connected with the *tortoise ?* The lady is thin, rather ashy yellow hair, a taking little hat. They are both in the prime of life. The children are eight and nine, a boy and a girl, a bright red dress, the boy a sailor suit, he has 'S.M.S.*Iltis'* on his cap. *A big steamer,* they are taken aboard, parting. *The gentleman goes aboard*—I cannot distinguish the country—a port like Amsterdam—' leave me alone with Rotterdam ' (to the voice on the left). One of them is speaking Dutch—as if it were *a journey round the world*—did not part with it—"

Tischner : " Who did not part with it ? "

" The fair-haired gentleman did not part with the object—*he can wear it on a ribbon on his chest.* Now I see the gentleman in his study—darkly furnished, a *greenish-black writing-table, broad without a top,* a pile of papers bound in yellow, in yellow envelopes on it—a bronze tray to his right, vases on the table, a kind of Roman vase—bronzed, black arabesques, a small urn— *a pen-tray made of some black material like stone*—a very pretty lamp on a stand by the side of the writing-table —a lamp-shade with pearls—*a book-case to his left,* next the door—*dull green unpolished*—he says *some Greek words* which I cannot repeat—can't be—I understand ' Euphrosyne ', before it ' Aganoia, Euphronesis '—I see the back of the tortoise again—like a lid, like a beautiful bowl—it lies there under the book-case as if it had no value, although it looks very valuable. He must be a tremendous idealist, truly a man of ideals. ' Therefore drink from this source of life, and the darkness and the light shall reflect themselves in thee.' Now I see a frame, in this frame a golden background from which a bronze head stands out, it hangs in the room, and is connected with this gentleman—it is strange how everything has bronze-coloured reflections to-day—this man was in India. I am made to think of Buddha—the lady has just been with him, in a tea-gown, he does not seem pleased with this, rings on her hands—*rings, sapphires and ruby—one like a sapphire*— her christian name is ' E., Edith, Elizabeth ', the one on the left says, ' Don't make hocus-pocus out of a steamer trip on the Rhine '. . . I will give you a résumé of the whole thing now—I fancy the object was won in a foreign country, and was *a companion on his travels,* is connected with some animal. *He is fond of the object, it is dear to him, he values it,* it is connected with something I should like to find out. One of them calls to me *diploma, gift of honour for something special."*

G. writes : " The packet contained the ' Militärverdienstorden ', a Bavarian war decoration which I received during the war. We can consider the following facts if we wish to find any obvious connexions between what H. said and the fate of the medal or myself. I had the medal on me when my regiment was stationed in the Caucasus. Our uniform consisted of buff tropical suits, and often of light-coloured tropical helmets. I used all my leisure in Tiflis to study the tropical fauna. My wife was not present when we embarked and left the ship. We were then interned in Salonika for a long time. I wore a tropical suit, and came across Greeks very frequently. We often played with the tortoises in the camp ; there were a great many of them. So I did come from a hot country and came back by steamer, sailing right round Europe. The writing table in my study is very broad and has a flat top, the pen-tray is as H. described it. Mrs. Gruber has a ring with a very beautiful sapphire. The statements, ' can be worn on a ribbon—diploma—gift of honour for some special thing,' may refer to the war medal."

We can take the experiment as positive ; the mention of the tortoises, the Greek words, and the gift of honour are particularly striking. I should particularly like to draw attention to the statement " he can also wear the ribbon on his chest," which apparently has no connexion with the statements directly preceding and following it. *Positive.*

119*th Experiment.* Object (unknown) : a box containing a bronze medal with the figure of a man on it, on the other side there was an inscription on it; it was about the size and shape of the oval metal checks given to the soldiers. T. gives H. the parcel.

" *Coins,* it has to do with foreign *coins, a locket—* a jubilee—this means nothing—I see *bronze* every now and again—*like the checks the wounded* have—what is this on a narrow main road ?—there is a *foreign coin in here, with an inscription*—but I can't read what is on it—I don't accept all this till I actually see it in visions—*military reviews, decorations* are being pinned on, all soldiers—*bronze medals* again and again—now he calls to me, ' but it is silver.' "

The experiment is interrupted, and the box put on one side. Another experiment, the 120th, is tried, then the box is taken up again, but no decisive statements are forthcoming; H. sees war pictures, troops, marching, columns, etc., so we put an end to it.

Gruber says that there might be a barely possible connexion with visions of troops, etc., as the image on the medal was that of a friend of his who fell in August, 1914, in Lorraine.

The result was positive as far as the recognition of the material and the shape is concerned. *Half positive.*

120*th Experiment.* Object (unknown) : a poem. *Negative.*

SITTING OF 11TH JULY, 1920

In H.'s flat. Present : Mrs. H., H., Gruber, and I.

121*st Experiment.* Object (unknown) : a small pen-knife belonging to Mrs. Gruber.

" Several voices—one says ' yellow, chased '—the second : ' this is bluff, it is the same bronze thing again '—the first says, ' mosaic.' *A girl in her teens is standing in front of a looking-glass with her hair down. She is brushing and combing it* ; behind her sits a *sculptor and models* the whole scene.—' Olympia !'—what does that mean ?—Something from Greece ?—No . . . A regatta : this is awful, I see them jump out of the boats into the water and swim. The feeling that something disagreeable is connected with it, *it has seen sad times.* Someone with frozen feet—again *a regatta,* a wonderful summer day, like the lake of Treptow, in the Mark (North Germany), *a great many sailing boats,* everything is white, clouds of dust ; how strange, so much smoke, is this fog or what is it?—rows of cut corn? Suddenly a room, a mahogany writing-table, a pale youngish lady, without a hat, in front of it, *her hair is parted in the middle, not drawn tightly,* large brown eyes. *Loneliness, longing, homesickness, restlessness, also bodily weakness, a feeling of weariness— longing for the children*—again the child standing in front of the glass, brushing and combing her hair— half-sisters? I don't know. They meet again, that is certain—it is connected with the pale brunette, *in the arms of a big fair man in uniform, flush of emotion, welcoming scene, dried up tears—again a sailing-boat,* but not in North Germany this time, now *here in the Alpine region,* I should almost like to say Starnberg— both in travelling clothes—it seems to me that they are husband and wife—they might be brother and sister—that one, a gentleman with a black cape, is here again, a soldier's coat with pleats, very sympathetic face, pointed beard, steel-blue eyes, short hair standing up, whiskers—a very thin nose—a Red Cross sister is connected in some way with him—*this girl must be a wild little thing, a school-girl,* now she sings ' Eia-popeia'. *A whirlwind, a ne'er do well.* Now I suddenly see *a clearing in a wood, tall fir-trees in a triangle, in front of it a large sloping field, a white house, two-storied*—I see the painter and the child go into it—this is not true."

Gruber says : " The italicized statements can be brought into connexion with the following events in Mrs. Gruber's life : after the end of the war Mrs. Gruber went to Switzerland to try to pick up a little in health and in hopes that it would relieve her state of mental depression a little. I was more or less lost in the Near East at the time. Our children remained in Munich. I came back in July, 1919, when we were able to have a happy meeting. My wife and I have sailed a great deal on the lake of Constance, on the shores of which my father has his country seat, which H. described very well indeed from his vision : a light-coloured two-storied house in a clearing at the top end of a big field. Our eldest daughter is a very lively and restless school-girl ; she was modelled two years ago. Neither H. nor Dr. Tischner knew any of these things."

This experiment can be considered as positive, as there are such surprising connexions between the data obtained from the object and events in the life of the owner ; the most remarkable thing seems to be the mention of the modelling of the child, a thing so very unexpected to a man of H.'s mode of life. *Positive.*

122nd and 123rd Experiments. Objects (unknown). *Negative.*

The objects were a parcel and a poem respectively.

SITTING OF 20TH JUNE, 1920

In H.'s flat. Present : Dr. von Hattingberg, who is a nerve specialist in Munich, H., and I.

It is first stated in the record that H. says he has had a heart attack, and is not feeling well.

124th and 125th Experiments. Object (unknown). *Negative.*

We could find no connexion between H.'s statements and the objects.

126th Experiment. Object (unknown) : a packet containing a coin with a date which Hattingberg had received from his fiancé on the day of their formal engagement. I handed it to H.

" *I see a young lady laying a large table, she puts the best napkins on the table, boards are put into the middle to lengthen it, the tablecloth is of a very fine damascus linen, flowers and stands.* The guests sit down, it is either *an engagement or a wedding, it does not look enough like a wedding. The bride is certainly dressed in white, a very airy garment . . .*"

T. " Can you describe anything more ? "

" They call out ' chemistry ' to me—*Lisbeth*—now it stops again, now a bracelet plays a part . . ."

I do not publish the remainder of the record, as nothing more fitted the object.

Hattingberg exchanged these dated coins with his fiancé on the day of their engagement, when they had a party to celebrate the occasion ; the table was oval, and leaves were put in to lengthen it. It was nicely laid in the manner described ; they were a fairly large party, and the fiancé's mother, who was generally called Lisbeth by the family, was present. H. clearly stated that it was an engagement by saying it was not enough like a wedding. No further connexions could be traced with the bracelet and what followed. I must mention in connexion with the remark about chemistry that H. had seen a chemical laboratory in the previous experiment, which was negative. Tischner tried to encourage him, as nothing more was forthcoming, and must have put him on to a wrong track. At any rate the experiment was decidedly positive. *Positive*.

SITTING WITHOUT THE COMMISSION

Present : H. and I. I had brought three little boxes packed exactly alike ; I had packed them myself.

127th Experiment. Object (unknown). *Negative*.

128th Experiment. Object (unknown) : an Egyptian scarab with hieroglyphics engraved on it.

" Something metallic," shall I say *antique*, it does not come from a numismatologist—I only see a black wall in front of me. It has disappeared, nice filigree work. *So dark, like in dark passages, deeper and deeper.* I see something like hewn stone in a sort of mine, but I probably concluded this as I only saw stone. Scales of thin metal. Not cuff links, are they ? "

Tischner : " No."

" I see the number ' 5 '. A dish like a full-moon, with filigree, the plate is yellow. *Something with strange letters, signs engraved on it. It certainly is antique, this is certain. It is antique, engraved, quite another age.*

Sandals, something like Jewish priests, strange priests, wearing coloured garb. Palaces at the time of the Roman Empire. The Orient, Orient. I see such foreign signs, I fancy they are Hebrew, *I cannot read them. A find, an antique find."*

It is quite obvious what is correct and what is not. It is not surprising that he should have taken Egyptian for Jewish priests. The darkness he refers to may be the passages to the tombs where the scarab may have been found. *Positive.*

After the next experiment H. told me that during the whole of the second experiment he could not help thinking of a scarab which he had worn on a ring which his sister subsequently wore on her watch-chain ; he had not dared to mention it. I am quite convinced that this statement is true, but of course it is of no scientific value. H. said that he was so annoyed with himself for not mentioning it that he had not been able to concentrate on the third object.

129th Experiment. Negative.

SITTING OF 29TH SEPTEMBER, 1920

In H.'s flat. Present : Dr. Recknagel, H., his friend Mr. M., and I.

130th Experiment. (Nearly) Negative.

SITTING ON THE EVENING OF 5TH OCTOBER, 1920

At H.'s flat. Present : Mrs. H., H., Professor Gruber, and I.

131st and 132nd Experiments. Negative.

133rd Experiment. Object (unknown) : a packet containing a little white frame like a locket, with a photo of a man.

Dr. Recknagel had left a sealed packet at the end of the last sitting. H. produced this with the seals untouched, and said that he had had the following dream about its contents :

EXPERIMENTS

" *A photo in a small frame*, like the picture of a child ; then *like a man*, then again a child, then it did not seem like a photo in a frame any more, but as a *locket.*"

I drew Recknagel's attention to the fact that it could not be considered as absolutely conclusive in the strictest sense, but as it was so similar in its results to other experiments done under the most stringent conditions, I thought it could be taken as positive. *Positive.*

134th Experiment. Object (unknown) : a key in a packet. *Negative.*

135th Experiment. Object (unknown) : packet containing a whistle. *Negative.*

The key and the whistle had been chosen for a special purpose. I wanted to obtain direct statements or descriptions of objects obtained by clairvoyance, so I had asked Gruber to choose quite ordinary things, without any particular historical or other associations. Now it is interesting to see that no attempt at a description of the object and no correct data from its history were obtained ; but why should not anything be said about the history of a key ? Whether this is due mainly to chance or to some deeper underlying cause is an open question.

136th Experiment. Object (unknown) : a packet containing a wooden cigarette box with a red and gold enamel pennant on it.

" A single post with a wreath round it. Then first of all *two children on the lawn*, pillars as if taken from a box of bricks—the children also have other toys, animals, the post began by being pretty large, then small with a green spiral on it. The children again are *carrying flowers in their hands*—now I see *a railway train* rolling along—what ? *Liliput ?—what sort of little flag ?* I must reject that thing about the Christmas Tree—I see a summer landscape—I only see *toys—a train, a toy* tied with a golden string—*little golden tinsel flags*—a whole set of children's toys—they don't call out anything to me to-day—I keep on seeing two children, *a boy and a girl*—now they are playing with *slides, like magic-lantern slides,* which you can keep turning round—' cheer up, you will only have to write three letters to-morrow '—now I see little ' Hinkels ' [1] *chicks,* now a middle-sized person like a *cook, she has something in her apron, the children come running up, they are delighted, she seems to have kittens* or chickens." (Pause.) " Now I see a large *lens, a large thing to look through* . . ." (Pause.) " Now I see a small pond where the children let their gold-fish swim."

Gruber says the cigarette box was a sailing prize, which he had won on the lake of Constance while staying at his father's house. H. mentions the pennant on it, the visions of playing children, the person bringing the kittens in her apron, the thing like a kaleidoscope, and the little train. The life of the family of Professor Gruber at Lindenhof, the family estate, circles round the children. They had a little train ; a kaleidoscope and a kitten were given to them ; the hens ran about all round the house. A number of indications of correct scenes without any attempt to combine them by intellectual processes. This experiment must be considered positive, though not one of the best. *Positive.*

SITTING OF 12TH OCTOBER, 1920

At H.'s flat. Present : Mrs. H., H., Mrs. and Miss Recknagel, and I.

137th and 138th Experiments. Negative.

These two experiments were again made with quite simple objects. The purpose was the same as in Nos. 134 and 135. The objects were a small blue glass ball and a key ; the descriptions did not fit the objects. H. said that the things chosen by Dr. Recknagel had

---

[1] *Gockel, Hinkel and Gakeleia* is the title of a delightful book by Clemens Brentano, about the adventures of a cock, a hen, and a chicken. " Hinkel " was the chicken.

very little "od" and had no action on him, so I did not ask Dr. Recknagel to attend the experiments again.

SITTING OF 16TH OCTOBER, 1920

In my sitting room. Present : H. and I.

139th Experiment. Object : a locket on a chain. I handed H. the parcel as usual. A student who lives in my house and was ill in bed at the time made the parcel. I knew the contents. The student could not influence H. in any normal way ; H. did not know him, but only knew it came from him.

" I see the object and not its history. An elliptical thing on a white background—*something rather like a chain—rolled up. A fine thin chain rolled up into an ellipse.* I do not see a bracelet, and don't want to come to that conclusion by that association. Something like a *small tablet* or like a stone . . ."

I asked him to draw the object. He drew a circle. The circle was not very round, as it had been drawn quickly ; it was 1·1 inch by 1 inch, the locket 1·1 inch. The object was known to me, but I was thinking of its history, not of its description. *Positive.*

140th Experiment. Object : the packet contained a small Indian figure made of brownish jasper or chalcedony. The details of the face and the folds of the garment were very clean-cut and hard.

" Something metallic, *with sharp edges.* I should almost like to say that it has the shape of a flower. I know it is wrong but it almost makes me think that it is an inkstand, but it is not one. It is not made of glass, *something that one puts on the table, an ornament, but it can be used as well.* Yes, it is an inkstand, silvery grey. The longer I look the more it condenses into a *figure,* made of metal. Looks like a *small bust* ; I sense it as if it were *sharp, a figure with sharp corners.* I see Beethoven, Mozart, Goethe—*a broad head.* But I also *see flowers.* The sharpness is most irritating. *With very sharp contours.* I can't make out whether it is old or new. Not plaster of Paris, something metallic."

It belongs to the student ; I had not told this to H. He supposed it must be so, and it put him out considerably, as he mentioned later on (see below). The head is broad and heavy. The student used it as a letter weight. *Positive.*

We got up after this experiment, and were standing in front of a small picture, when one of H.'s alternations of personality occurred and " Beethoven " spoke through him. He said that the " spirits " had said the words " Buddha Indian statuette " several times to H. It was such a pity that H. had not repeated it. It would be a thousand times better for him to say things which did not fit the objects than to suppress correct information ; I was to tell him that.

Thereupon Beethoven withdrew, and H.'s normal personality returned. He asked me what had happened and confirmed the fact that he had thought of an Indian figure, but he thought it most improbable that the student should have such a figure. He said that he would rather have bitten off his own tongue than have divulged that to me.

I want to report this as being of considerable psychological interest to people who are familiar with the phenomena of dissociation of personality ; they will know what an impression of genuineness this gives.

SITTING OF 23RD NOVEMBER, 1920

In H.'s flat. Present : Mrs. H., H., Gruber, and I.

141*st Experiment.* Object : the packet contained a club badge like an escutcheon shaped tie-pin. It had an ice-axe and a coiled rope engraved on it, so that they showed up in gilt on a black enamel background ; two skis appear, projecting obliquely from behind it at the top and bottom.

" I am being influenced banefully from the outside, it is by my friend Müller. He says that no single experiment will succeed. I began by seeing some *painting on glass*, as small as on a *tie-pin, like inlaid work*, certainly something *painted*—as if there were little chips of stone artificially put together. I see two little hands holding the object as if they wanted to fix it—as if a photo were painted on it ; how odd it is *this small round thing, something which pricks, like a stalk."*

The needle is neither painted nor mosaic, but the enamel on it looks as if it were. The needle was clearly recognized. *Positive.*

142*nd Experiment.* Object : a small straightened piece of a copper shell-ring, packed up in the usual way. It was handed to H. at 9.41 p.m.

9.43. " I am being fooled, I can see nothing but *smoke—ploughed up holes, like when shells strike the ground.* I see volcanic *eruptions, I see fumes—tremendous fumes. I saw when it struck down there, flew to pieces in the air, I even saw aeroplanes dropping bombs ;* low houses, *like in the mountains, as if it were hilly.* I see a *dug-out,* a low white building, and a great many uniforms. As if a regimental staff were there. There is so much going to and fro. I see dug-outs half torn up. *It is certainly connected with the war. A war scene is* before the eye of my mind. Now the object is somewhere else. *It lies on a primitive wooden table. I see it twisted like this*—(holding his hand bent) *not flat like in there. It lies on the wooden table. There are only men about."*

T. : " What do the men look like ? "

" Men with long hair and long beards, rather dirty. I can't quite grasp the situation. There are hardly any people in the district and yet there are low houses, bad roads, a great many crusts on the main roads. I see carts with small horses." 9.55.

The shell-ring was picked up by Gruber in the Vosges and used as a letter-weight in his dug-out. Gruber says, "It was a piece of a copper guiding-ring which had been straightened out subsequently. I found it in the Vosges where my company was entrenched. The description given of the exploding shell might relate to the experience of the object or to my own. I used it as a letter-weight on plain white tables in many dug-outs." *Very Positive.*

143rd Experiment. Negative.

144th Experiment. Object : the packet contained Mrs. Gruber's passport. The experiment was begun at (H. was in a trance) :

10.42. " A silver plate, *with engraved letters,* form tabular with a sign engraved on it. I can't make out what it is—a memento ! "

Gruber : " Can you tell me who it belongs to ? "

10.52. " I think *it belongs to your wife."*

H. comes out of trance ; there is a pause, then he begins again :

" Dedication, memento with dedication engraved on it, at any rate *a mark of recognition. Rectangular shape."*

German passports are little rectangular books with a dull brown cover on which is stamped the Prussian Eagle, and an inscription in relief. This forms a round medal-like relief in the middle. The pages on the inside are green.

The only positive statements concern the inscription, the owner and the shape of the object. The expression " mark of recognition " can be taken as a paraphrase of the word passport. It is so characteristic that we can consider the experiment as positive, although so few details and facts were mentioned. *Positive.*

SITTING OF 5TH DECEMBER, 1920

At Professor Gruber's. Present : Mrs. Gruber, Mr. C. von Salis, Gruber, H., and I.

145th Experiment. (Known to Mrs. G. and to Salis.) Object : a packet containing Mr. von Salis' signet ring.

H. found the new surroundings rather disturbing, and only proceeded to choose a packet after getting used to them. We were sitting at a round table.

5.45 p.m. H. takes the small box and puts it back again. He chooses another.

5.48. " I begin by seeing a little bunch of dried pansies ; now I see absolutely nothing more."

Tischner puts H. into light hypnotic trance.

5.55. " Now I see a ring in the first box."

He takes up the second box.

" I do not see the ring any more now that I have this in my hand."

Gruber gives H. the first box.

" I see an elderly couple ; what is the matter to-day ? *It is an object which must have passed through many hands.* An elderly and a younger couple in travelling clothes standing in front of a shop window—indefinite, indefinite ; it is all jumbled up—I don't know why I see the elderly couple—I see a ring on the elderly lady's hand. First of all pretty thick with a stone, now an excrescence is forming, pointed at the top, seems to be dark blue like a sapphire—I have so few ideas to-day— I saw a young couple in light clothes in front of a shop window in a foreign town. I fancy that the young people have travelled to the place where the elder ones live— *the object must have changed hands several times.* It is certainly *a present given to the young people by elderly persons*—it is getting twisted into the form of an old-fashioned circlet, *like a small crown, with teeth like this.*"

H. makes a gesture as if he were drawing a few short diverging lines in the air with his finger.

" I still see it *in the form of a ring*—now they are showing me all kinds of rings—*the elderly people and the younger are related to one another.* The elderly lady is thin, bony, frail, pale—they tell me that *there is a ring inside the parcel.*"

The experiment is quite positive. The signet-ring was inherited by Mr. von Salis years ago from his deceased grandmother. The statement that he sees the ring with an excrescence, like a sapphire, is strange, as Mrs. Gruber was wearing one with a large sapphire on that evening. It is not possible to tell whether H. saw that ring consciously or not. *Positive.*

146*th Experiment. Negative.*

147*th Experiment.* Object (known to Gruber) : a packet containing the photo of Mrs. Gruber and her daughter, in a frame.

" I keep on seeing *a family picture with children,* I see a small *photo with children,* like a ladder, arranged like organ-pipes. *I have the sensation of holding a photo in my hand.* I refuse to accept the remainder, but I can't get past it . . . *There is a Picture in here."* *Positive.*

148*th Experiment.* Object (known to Mrs. Gruber). *Negative.*

SITTING OF 15TH DECEMBER, 1920

At Mrs. T.'s. Present : Mrs. Schn, Mrs. T., Miss M., Mr. Tr., Mr. T., H., and I.

149*th Experiment.* Object (known to Mrs. Schn) : the packet contained a large mother-of-pearl shell mounted on a wire stand. Mrs. Schn had packed it.

I handed it to H.

" The object *was taken from* your *writing-table."* (Tischner's.)

H. can't get on. He stands up and sits down in a corner of the room. He said that the gentleman who had just arrived put him out, and he would go on with the experiment in this corner. So we both of us sat there for the next two experiments ; the others could not tell what was said till I read out the record of the experiment.

" Made of clear white glass, as transparent as glass, not an inkstand : it must be a present, it is not an article of common use. It gives me the impression of coming from the *sea, it has its origin in the water.* I see it in a gentleman's hand, he brings it back from a journey. I keep on *seeing water. As if prismatic rays came from the object, it is irridescent, and reflects different colours.*"

The two halves of the shell were connected by a small hinge so that they formed a sort of small box. The object did come from a writing-table, but not from mine ; it had stood on the writing-table of Mrs. Schn's father. I could not find out anything more about its fate. It did shine very decidedly in different colours. *Positive.*

150*th Experiment.* Object (known to Dr. and Mrs. Tischner) : the little heart-shaped bowl mentioned in Experiment No. 79.

" *It is made of metal,* gives the impression of being some sign or badge. Like bronze, colour darkish yellow, shape rounded—(this conclusion perhaps by guess-work)—a round medallion. *A large room with people in festive garb.* Why this so suddenly. *I see Mrs. Tischner among them, the gentlemen in dress-clothes, but there are some people in fantastic dress*—perhaps because we just talked of the carnival. It was worn or *given at a fête. A gentleman with a key or a silver tray.*"

H. wants to break off the experiment, so I tell him that a great deal is correct to encourage him.

" *It is connected with Mrs. Tischner, it is handed to her.* Madam, you are decorated, but not by the man who carries the tray, by someone else. It keeps on reminding me of Professor Gruber's Ski-club badge, but it is *nobler,* a mark of honour, a decoration, *but it is connected with the ceremony, as if to fix it in the memory.*"

The fantastic costumes might apply to the Polish villagers who were present at the wedding. *Positive.*

SITTING OF 16TH DECEMBER, 1920

At Dr. Richter's. Present : Count Klinkowström, Dr. Richter, H., and I.

TELEPATHY AND CLAIRVOYANCE

151st–154th Experiments. Negative.
I met H. in the street on the way to Dr. Richter's. He was from the first very much upset by the new surroundings and the new faces.

SITTING OF 14TH JANUARY, 1921

In H.'s flat. Present : Gruber, H., and I.
155th Experiment. Object (unknown) : a sealed parcel containing a flint axe-head packed tightly in a cardboard box. It had been sent to Gruber by a friend in the Engadine (by the translator).

" Frightfully cold, I see dark water, it must be something strange, I see so many people. *The object must come from a foreign land*, from the East ; Eastern climate, I *can feel the cold*. It almost seems to me to be Asia—Siberia, rather like a fish, ' tortoisy.' Impression of a cross. I again see uniforms, foreign ones, I see men with fairly long beards, *primitive, it points to a primitive country.* When you came (to Gruber) the word (China) was called out to me, but I have not got the perception of anything Chinese—I conclude it must be Eastern Russia. They keep on calling ' weapon' to me, foot-warmer. Saint on small pedestal ? ? I don't seem to get any further.—I see such a distorted face—*it does not come from the Gruber family, not an heirloom*—either *it is a find which did not take place in Germany*, or it is something brought in by the war, at any rate *it is not a present made in a conventional way. Something made in a foreign land* ; I caught a glimpse of a Russian priest's head with a long beard. Frightful cold emanates from it."

An attempt at crystal-gazing was unsuccessful. H. sees absolutely nothing.

" *I don't see any connexion with the Gruber family at all*—I keep on seeing large black waves spurting up, very monotonous—I incline to think that it contains a work of plastic art."

The object was put aside. Another experiment, No. 156, was tried, at the end of which the parcel was taken up again.

"A frosty feeling emanates from it, again black water, a black sea. The East, *The Stone Age*, something *stoned* (not fossilized, nor turned to stone, ' Versteint '). They call out ' Neptune ' to me. Statue of Neptune, the object is connected with water, *came in a ship across the sea*, perhaps a warship, as I caught a glimpse of a naval battle."

The flint axe-head dated from the Achulean period ; it had been found in the South of England. The experiment was decidedly positive, as the object was quite out of the scope of guessing, or conclusion by probabilities. The most remarkable statements are those about a primitive country, the sensation of cold, and the words " the East ", " Siberia ", as Europe then probably had much the same character as Siberia nowadays.

Translator's comment : I was given the axe-head by a cousin of mine in England. It was chipped. He said it had been found in a quarry somewhere in the New Forest. Hearing of my friend Gruber's experiments, I packed it very tightly in a small cardboard box, wrapped this up in strong brown paper, tied it up with string in the usual way, crosswise, and sealed it. I was in the Engadine at the time, and only mentioned the fact to my wife and to another lady, neither of whom would have communicated the contents ; besides they promised not to do so. They none of them knew H. My wife knows Gruber. I gave the parcel to a brother-in-law saying it was to be sent to Gruber unopened, but not saying anything more about it. So no one in Munich knew anything about it. I had written to Gruber that I was sending him a parcel for H., and asked him to ask H. to say as much as possible about the history of the object, and not to be in a hurry to open it. I also asked him to send me a report of the experiment. I expected the experiment to take place within a few days of sending it, and had quite forgotten about it by the time the experiment actually did take place. *Positive.*

156th *Experiment.* (Object known to Gruber.) Object : A bronze medallion, a ski-ing prize won by Gruber at Weissen See in the Vosges, in the usual packet.

" A thin woman's arm—seems to be very massive, like a bracelet—now I see pieces put together—it is made of separate parts, with foreign designs among them—I first of all saw the hand without a bracelet— with a ring like a snake, then a bracelet, with scales in close rows—then I saw the lady feeding goats with the selfsame hand—*a country house in a mountainous district*, a fence behind the house—behind this fence goats are being fed—it is something intimate, with a meaning—so it is a present all the same—*a memento*— they call out French-Switzerland to me—*an old gentleman with a beard like Kaiser Wilhelm*—striped trousers, a white waistcoat, and a black tail-coat—a dark blue tie, with a pearl in it, a high collar with rounded corners, he wears a signet-ring, it seems to be an aquamarine, and a wedding-ring next to it. *The gentleman is at least at the end of the sixties, grey beard—middle-sized*—he is in the same house, now I see him on the first floor—it has a shell-shaped balcony—the gentleman is on the balcony, wears glasses—seems old and kind—he waves his hand to those below—I see the hens coming out of the stable—I think I hear the name ' Emma '—now I am on a sailing yacht—*there must be water in the neighbourhood, a pond or little lake*, with a small sailing-boat on it. It is not a bracelet."

The lake and, perhaps, French-Switzerland are positive, as the lake is in the French-speaking part of the Vosges. The description reminds me strongly of the gentleman who gave away the prizes. The other data cannot be checked. *Slightly positive.*

157th Experiment. Object (known) : a small box tied up with string containing a hundred rouble note.

Tischner puts H. into a slight trance.

" It makes me laugh when I take the object in my hand."

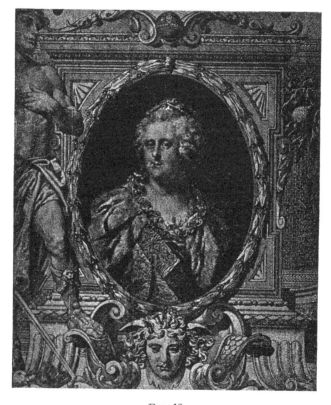

FIG. 18.

Trance, during which H. says a good many things which have nothing to do with the object. H. wakes up.

" It makes me laugh, it is connected with the carnival—a Prussian glove dipped in French blood— I see something like a bird of paradise's feathers, *Lady's head-dress*—the head-dress is built up on a head-band—a brunette in a reddish-violet dress—*like a Rubens figure.*"

Trance, in which a very erotic personage, the Marquess of Tourcoing, appears; he speaks pretty fluent French to Mrs. H. H. comes out of trance.

" I see *a head, a Rubens female figure with a diadem and a feather—it is on something on an oval mount,* but many coloured : *a picture of some object.* As if there were *women's heads in it in Rubens' style, full, fresh women's heads.*"

I asked H. to draw what he had described ; he did so. He began by drawing a square frame.

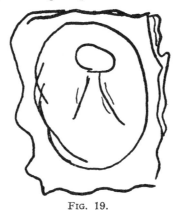

FIG. 19.

Gruber said : " I thought that the frame was oval ? " —so as to try to mislead him.

" *The oval is inside.*"

While he was drawing I expressed surprise that he did not draw a rectangular frame with straight lines.

He said that there were ornaments on the outside.

The hundred rouble note had the head of Catherine II of Russia on it. There was another head of the same Czarin as a water mark, so H. was quite right when he mentioned several women's heads. There is a diadem on the picture, this seems to have been the first thing seen. We can hardly put it down to chance that the top line of the rectangle should have been drawn the straightest, as a figure cuts into the frame on the left-hand side : in fact its curvature approximately follows the line of the leg, there is an ornament cutting into the frame on the lower side, and the ornament at the top of the right-hand side is slightly indicated. The statement that it has lively colours is correct in so far as the hundred rouble note has orange striation and the design in black on a yellow background. There is green, brown, red, and violet on the back of the note. H. seems to have got an impression of the object the picture describes, as he says : " It is of something " and " a picture of some object ". *Decidedly positive.*

SITTING OF 19TH JANUARY, 1921

In Gruber's house. Present : a lady, three gentlemen, Mrs. Gruber, Dr. Richter, Gruber, H., and I.

Both Gruber and I found that H. was very much put out by the new faces. One of the gentlemen especially distracted his attention so much that we had to ask him to leave the sitting subsequently. So the first experiments were carried out under very unfavourable conditions, H. making a great many statements, of which very few bore any relation to the subject ; this is quite in accordance with what I said on page 94 ; it leads us to conclude that quite apart from chance there is some definite factor concerned which is not always present when it is wanted.

158th–159th Experiments. Negative.

160th Experiment. Object : a packet containing a prayer book bound in ornamented imitation leather.

" There is something mineral about it without a doubt. Something dark, like a brass plate with an inscription."

Pause, in which the 159th experiment was taken up again without success.

" Now I perceive that it is a book *bound in leather, in some sort of book-lover's edition.* A black stone with an inscription—volume of *book-lover's edition.*"

I think we can take this experiment as positive, as the book is described very characteristically. *Positive*.

161st *Experiment*. Object (unknown) : a packet containing a lock of hair.

" *Small pin, like a safety-pin, like a buckle—very thin like a small bow. It is a buckle with a needle on it, like this.*"

Makes a drawing.

" *Buckle was worn on a belt or a tie*, with a stone in the middle, I see it on a pale yellow belt, also on a tie *from a lady*. Between thirty and forty years old."

Gruber, thinking the lock had been cut off long ago, asked the owner, a girl of nineteen, whether anything had been kept with it : he said nothing about the result of the experiment. The young lady said that she used to wear a buckle just on the lock of hair she had cut off, and showed it to Gruber. It was just like the one H. had drawn, as I was able to see for myself. As it often happens that the object itself is not described, but that events out of its history are related, these data cannot be put down to chance, and the experiment must be considered positive. *Positive*.

162nd *Experiment*. Object (unknown) : a packet containing a small rosary, the beads of which were little roses. It had a heart on it as a pendant.

" Red, heart-shaped, *like petals of a rose*. Again stuck on paper." *Positive*.

SITTING OF 24TH FEBRUARY, 1921

In my flat. Present : H. and I.

I took advantage of a visit from H., who came to see me on some business, to try an experiment.

163rd *Experiment*. Object : a packet containing a small Egyptian figure, made of brown pottery.

" Like an oval vase, something longish, not glass, has coloured reflections, *might be earthenware*, it is not coloured glass, *brownish*, at any rate it is a vessel, flowers could be put into it, but I don't wish to imply that it is a vase. No ! It is more like an antique vessel, I hear the word ' majolica ', transfused with blue, an oval vessel, Greece, *it has certainly come across the seas.* A mineral which has crystallized in the sea, which has lain in the sea, *or come across the sea. I caught a glimpse of a pleasure steamer coming across the Mediterranean. A lady who bought this thing as a souvenir of a distant country,* perhaps not intending to give it to you at all. *The influence of a lady still adheres to the object, she is still living,* I can't quite distinguish her. *Has quite a peculiar turn of mind, and all the same she is rather robust and dry.''*

A lady bought the object in Egypt ; she passed through Athens on her return journey. It is not a present to me. The characteristics of the lady are very well given, the dryness especially is quite typical. H. knew the lady in question, but there was nothing which could lead him to believe that the object was in any way connected with her. If he had by any chance been led to identify her, he could have described her appearance and her character much more precisely. This makes me think that he perceived these characteristics without a vision of any particular person. *Positive.*

Sitting of 28th February, 1921

At H.'s flat. Present : Dr. von Hattingberg, H., and I.

164th Experiment. Object (unknown). *Negative.*

165th Experiment. Object : Hattingberg had packed the medal mentioned in experiment No. 126 (presented at his engagement) in the long cardboard case of a violin bow.

The experiment was quite negative. H.'s statements were all influenced by the case the bow was packed in, for instance he alluded to a roll of parchment, a doll's sunshade, an arrow, a snake-skin, a violin bow. He said himself that he was afraid that all this was due to guesswork. On discussing the experiment later on with Hattingberg, we both came to the conclusion that the results were not due to wilful guesswork, as any imposter who was at all cunning would have suspected a trap, and not let himself be deceived by the mode of packing. H. must have let himself be led on by the natural associations suggested by the case. *Negative.*

166*th Experiment.* Object : Hattingberg's wedding-ring.

While H. and I were talking, Hattingberg, who had seated himself at another table where we could not watch him, slipped off his wedding-ring, and put it in the case used in the previous experiment.

" It is nothing at all—there is something pointed in it like a corkscrew, I can't identify it, like a pencil, I see something silvery—middle-sized, they call out '*ring*' to me, but I can't accept that, I see a longish form, about the size of an index, there is a bend at the top of it, like the barb of a key, this sort of curve."

Designing it with his finger in the air.

" It is a small key, but I don't see it distinctly. I see it gleaming like silver, like a key. I am very much influenced by the case—they keep on calling to me '*Ring ! Ring !*' " *Positive.*

Neither Hattingberg nor I think that H. noticed the ring being taken off or missed it on Hattingberg's finger, as H. is a very poor observer. H. had sat with his eyes closed right away from Hattingberg during the whole of the experiment ; we could safely draw this conclusion, with a fair probability of its being correct. If he had noticed it and wanted to deceive us, he would have been much more emphatic about the ring. Of course, it might be a case of cryptomnesia, but this experiment fits into its place in the whole series so well that it hardly seems to require a different explanation.

H. felt decidedly ill in April, 1921 ; he also felt as if he had lost the gift of clairvoyance ; this feeling of course tended to spoil results. I tried two experiments with him, but both were unsuccessful.

167th–168th Experiments. Negative.

SITTING OF 11TH MAY

H. called on me, so we tried a few experiments.

169th Experiment. Object : the packet contained a button off a soldier's uniform.

" Shaped like a ring, *round, curved surface,* like a small brooch."

On my asking H. what he saw, he drew a flat segment of a circle. The button had a curved surface ; he had drawn it from the side. *Positive.*

170th Experiment. Object : a packet containing a small brooch made of Tula silver, with a pattern of small squares on it.

" I don't see anything at all, I see small squares, the object must have small squares."

H. can't get on any further. *Slightly positive.*

171st Experiment. Object : a packet containing a wedding-ring.

" Tortoiseshell."

As H. can get no further, I tell him that it is not tortoiseshell.

" ' Say *Ring* ' they call to me, *a gold ring, a thick wedding-ring.* Like a coat of arms, small lozenges."

H. went on to say things about a lady and gentleman at a railway station, and on steamers.

These statements were not characteristic, but were within the limits of probability.

The wedding-ring belonged to a gentleman whose wife was of aristocratic descent, so the statement about the coat of arms might be taken symbolically. The ring was a very thick one. *Positive.*

Out of six instances in which rings were contained in the parcels presented to H., he identified them five times. He hardly ever thought he saw a ring erroneously. This is a remarkable fact which can hardly be put down to chance.

TELEPATHY AND CLAIRVOYANCE

Present : H. and I.

172nd Experiment. Object : a packet containing half a buckle taken from a boy's belt ; there were some letters engraved on it.

"*Infantile feeling, as if a child were connected with it.*" H. goes on to speak of toys, etc., apparently conclusions by guessing, or associations which got mixed up with his perceptions. Then he ends up by saying : "There is a small brooch in it—*there is something written on it.*"

It at once strikes us that he immediately recognized that it was connected with a child. The rectangular plate of the buckle is rather like a brooch. *Slightly positive.*

173rd Experiment. Object : the parcel contained a small cardboard box with an animal embroidered on it in outline.

"*Quite green,* like a field. Like a picture-postcard, *I see something green.* It is not compact, it might be made of cloth or *paper. It is not a three-dimensional body.* Green gelatine or *green paper.* They tell me 'printed card ', but I don't accept that. *At any rate it is made of paper.* I have the feeling that there is nothing on it. It comes from a lady—as if something had been packed in it. It is not at all scented. Is like an entrance card, but is not one. A voice comes and says that sweets were packed in it, *it comes from a child.* They call out, '*Christmas ! Christmas ! Christmas !* '"

A child had done the embroidery on the box. Green was by far the most prevalent colour. When I asked its history, I was told that the box was a Christmas present. H. had dwelt several times on the main characteristic of the object, its being made of cloth or paper ; this he might have concluded from the lightness but he could not have concluded the other data by guesswork. *Positive.*

EXPERIMENTS

AUTUMN SITTING

Present : Dr. Gallinger, H., and I.

174th–175th Experiments. (Objects unknown.) *Negative.*

These last experiments were performed in the autumn of 1921, when H. was in bad health, and was already the subject of very strong inhibitions.

I want to describe just one more experiment with H., which is rather interesting from several points of view. I had asked H. and his secondary personalities, especially Richard Wagner, several times, whether we could not try to get H. to cryptoscopize objects and writing directly, but we had never actually proceeded to do so, till the middle of December, 1919, when I tried this several times, without success. I will not publish this series, which does not form part of the series of psychoscopic experiments, and which simply prove that H. did not possess that faculty.[1] I will just give one of them here as an example and because it is of some psychological interest.

176th Experiment. Object (unknown) : Envelope containing the number " 921 ".

I wanted to give H. the chance of considering the object for a longer time, so I left him an envelope with a number consisting of three digits which was unknown to me. I had wrapped it up in violet tissue paper, gummed the envelope, and stuck a number of gummed strips of paper with my name on them to make sure it was not opened. It was only meant to be a sort of preliminary test. I came back after a fortnight. H. told me, very sorrowfully, that he had not been able

---

[1] To prevent any possible misinterpretation I wish to state that I have recorded all the experiments on psychoscopy done with H. and none of those on telepathy and cryptoscopy. This does not detract from the value of my statistics, as it is well known that different mediums have different faculties, and that these must be kept separate if you really want to form a judgment on the medium.

The fact that H. had flashes of cryptoscopic faculty in certain circumstances and sometimes recognized the actual objects does not alter this.

to read the contents. A sudden change of personality took place and " Richard Wagner " said that H. did not possess the faculty of cryptoscopizing, that he was only able to perform experiments on psychoscopy such as we had been doing. The spirits could cryptoscopize, but had other things to do. However, to prove his statement he said that the number in the envelope was " 921 ". Personally, I am quite sure that H. did not open the envelope as he is an honest and reliable man, beside being so clumsy and childish that I don't think that he could have done it so neatly if he had tried. Of course, this experiment is of no scientific value, as it was not done under test conditions, but it is of considerable psychological interest. Mrs. H. told me " Richard Wagner " had told her three days before I came " H. need know nothing about it ; when Tischner comes I will tell him what it is ". In fact, a week before, " Richard Wagner " had told a friend of H.'s what the contents were. This may seem very odd to a layman, but these phenomena are well known to psychopathologists, and seem quite genuine to them.

I should like to add the reports of the few experiments which have been done with H. since the publication of the second edition. His health became worse and worse, so that we could rarely attempt any experiments.

SITTING OF 20TH SEPTEMBER, 1921

Present : the psychologist, Dr. Hoesch-Ernst, H., and I.

177th Experiment. Object (known to Tischner). *Negative.*

178th Experiment. Object (known to Mrs. H.-E.). I had given Mrs. H.-E. a small box, paper and string. She packed one of the usual small pocket-pencils with a ring at the end of it, in the next room. H. and I had no idea what she had chosen. She handed it to H.

" *Ring, pencil, pocket-pencil* ; a red stone, a birthday

present, I see the *ring* lying there, it is really only a wedding ring, but there is a red stone all the same. A voice says : ' not a ring.' "

You might say that the choice is not large when a lady packs an object ; a pencil and a ring would be among the things most probably chosen. But ladies often have all sorts of things at their disposal, such as keys, hair-pins, combs, mirrors, etc., especially if they come into town for the day. H. and I had expected her to have brought some specially selected things for the experiments. I should certainly not have guessed at so simple a thing. We might think that another thing which happened to be close by had been guessed. I think we can find another and more probable explanation. As mentioned above, the pencil had a ring at the end of it. This H. seems to have sensed, and to have expanded it in his imagination and built up on it. He often does that (see, for instance, the 172nd experiment), so it seems more likely that this should have been the case than that luck and successful guesswork were the true factors which led him to this result. *Positive.*

SITTING OF 5TH OCTOBER, 1921

At Tischner's. H. called, so we tried an experiment. Present : H. and I.

183rd Experiment. We tried an experiment, although H. was feeling very poorly. The result was negative. I only mention it for completeness' sake.

Chance should be independent of health, so that negative experiments in these circumstances tend to support the theory of the supernormal origin of clairvoyance, as shown by H. in his knowledge of the objects of former experiments.

Since then H. has been very ill, too ill for experiments.

More experiments on psychoscopy with other mediums may be recorded, besides Miss von B. and Mr. H. This faculty does not seem so rare. The next best series of experiments was obtained with a gentleman who unfortunately refused to allow me to publish them ; in fact he tore up the reports.

I will first describe an experiment with Mrs. W. She varied considerably in the power of her clairvoyant faculty, and I have most unfortunately lost part of the records.

179th Experiment. Object : a letter in an envelope.

I am leaving out the statements on character, as they tend to depend on subjective judgment as to their correctness, as opposed to the objective reality of the other data produced.

" I see the person connected with *copper,* could *that be hair with a metallic sheen* ? A lot of the work must be done in a stooping position or *leaning forward*— I see something being used which seems to be of the nature of a *small brush, the person has something in her hand, which is rather like a small brush,* I don't believe that this is symbolical. I fancy it is connected with the *person's work*—like a tooth-brush with five redmarks on the back. I also see a larger brush, *also a stand like those used to put blackboards on. A very large window, a great deal of light—rather a muddle, there seems to be a general mix-up, many different colours, might be a palate, particularly bright colours, green, red, blue, white, no black, she does not seem to care for it.* And yet so much black seems to appear all at once, a great black curtain drawn with force, ' all very black ' as if the room were transformed into a morgue. A coffin covered up with a cloth, but I see no corpse—perhaps *it is the funeral of one of life's great hopes,* either a great deal has been buried or this is yet to come. *Great pain,* a sort of woodenness coming over the person. *The favourite position seems to be leaning back with crossed legs,* suddenly a light seems to have gone out in him. *Blood blue,* not according to the familiar expression, I fancy impure blood, must have had inflammation of the veins."

EXPERIMENTS

The writer of the letter was a lady with red hair ; she is a painter. The brushes can probably be interpreted as paint brushes. The remainder of the description speaks for itself. The lady uses strong colours but never uses black. It was during her divorce that she wrote this letter, " a great deal has been buried," etc., might refer to that. Her characteristic attitude is very well described, she really has blue blood. The medium could not have any notion of what was in the envelope, nor was the author of the letter known to her. *Positive.*

Mrs. W. differs especially from H. in often having symbolical visions, which she recognizes as symbolical, and proceeds to interpret ; then in giving more detailed descriptions of character, Mrs. W. often used the expression "it appeared" ("es hat geheissen"). She answered our questions as to the nature of the perceptions which led to this statement, by saying that it was a perception midway between seeing and hearing. If I understood her explanation correctly, it must be that she hears the things at the same time as they appear to her in script, much in the same way as some people see colours when they hear certain tones in music.

I found a very clever medical student who was gifted in this way ; unfortunately, I was only able to do but a few experiments with him. One evening in the spring of 1920 I improvised a few experiments on the spur of the moment, one of which was psychoscopic.

180*th Experiment.* Object : a lady whom the gentleman only knew quite superficially handed him a ring she was wearing.

" An old town, the ring *comes from a gentleman* who wanted to become a *theologian.* He studied a good many other things as well, and met with a great deal of opposition. *He died at the age of* 54 *or* 64. *His wife was from the North.* I see Frisian blood, *she already had children.*"

The lady had to make inquiries before she could check these statements. A great many of them turned out to be correct. The gentleman was a theologian, but studied other subjects as well. He met with a great deal of opposition. He died at the age of 64, and his wife came from North Germany (we were not able to find out whether she was of Frisian origin) and had children from her first marriage.

181st *Experiment.* Object : another time a lady gave him a bracelet-watch with a locket on it.

" *Grail, a drama. The longing of one in exile.* Paradiesbett,[1] perhaps it hung there. Relationship. They have two kinds (of influence)."

T. : " How do you mean ? "

" *There are two kinds of radiations coming from it.* From her relations, envy from her aunt. *Then there is a lady friend. The ribbon was kissed.* It is of two kinds. I don't know, *this is a quiet friendship.* Half a year ago, August, September, of last year. *Theresienstrasse. A* tall *thin gentleman.* Perhaps it was bought there. *He looks as if he were 27 or 28, but he is older, perhaps* 35. *Light brown, black frock-coat.* Yes, yes, *Kissed.* Is there a picture in it ? "

Miss K : " There was."

" This bracelet previously passed through two people's hands, two ladies ; this was not the case with the watch. There is a funeral, a cemetery, funeral service, etc. One of them looks like Mrs. M. L. ; dressed in black."

The lady said that she had received the bracelet with the locket from a gentleman as a parting gift. She had played parts of Parsival to him out in the country, and had read Parsival and " The Mystery of the Grail " with him. Mr. R. had no friends at all ; he felt lonely, and longed for somebody who could sympathize with him. She suffered a good deal from the behaviour of her aunt during this friendship ; she put this down

---

[1] A German make of metal bedsteads.

to ill-will and envy on her aunt's part. A most intimate lady friend of hers was with her out in the country. Mr. R. wrote to her subsequently that he had kissed the bracelet ; it was pure friendship. The description of the gentleman answers that of her violin-master who used to live in the Theresienstrasse ; it is very good. He often wears a frock-coat, he was 34 when he gave her lessons, but looked much younger. The statement that the object passed through the hands of two ladies is true of the watch, but not of the bracelet. *Positive.*

182*nd Experiment.* Object : the lady mentioned in the 180th experiment handed him a cigarette-case, just as it was, not packed in any way.

" *The sea near Hamburg, or where Heligoland lies in front of it. A park. You have received it from a gentleman.* An idealist, a writer. *You have known the gentleman three years. Served as an officer.* Now I see the *Odeonsbar—Grünwald.*"

The lady had received the cigarette-case from a gentleman whom she had known three years ; it was given to her as a Christmas present in Bremen at a country house in a park. The gentleman was an officer at the time. The lady is a South German, and nothing could lead you to suppose that she or the object had any connexion with Bremen. There was no dedication or inscription on the cigarette-case which could have revealed this to the clairvoyant. I don't lay much stress on the Odeonsbar and Grünwald, as it is most natural that a cigarette-case in Munich should have been there.

We had one more sitting at Professor Gallinger's ; Professor Geiger, the philosopher, was present. We made two experiments with objects unknown to us, both of which were negative. Mr. S. had to be asked several times before he agreed to try, and then he was nervous and self-conscious. He told me himself that he was by no means in a suitable frame of mind at the time and that the feeling that something was expected of him prevented him from getting into it. This is a point which plays a great part in this kind of experiment, when conducted scientifically ; the more official the character of the investigation the less likely is it to bring good results. An experimenter who is known to be a hardened sceptic is hardly likely to have positive results at all.

I want to finish up this record with a few words about the Munich characterologist, Dr. Ludwig Aub, whose supernormal faculties seem to consist of a mixture of telepathy and clairvoyance. His characterological statements depend largely on physiognomical and graphological knowledge ; from these he proceeds to draw conclusions by deliberate association, and by what we might call intuitive perception. But some of his statements can only come from telepathy or clairvoyance. (p. 161.) Here are a few examples.

I had brought a gentleman to see Dr. Aub under a false name.

Dr. Aub did not go into the characterology of the gentleman, but began by describing his parents. Among other most descriptive statements, he said :

" Your mother " (she never lived in Munich, and Dr. Aub did not know her) " used to do very beautiful embroidery."

This was particularly interesting, and has the same value for me as the result of an exact experiment, because the gentleman had told me about ten minutes before, in the street, that his mother used to do some perfectly lovely work. We had not spoken at all in the waiting-room, so as not to give Dr. Aub any clues. This appears to have been quite characteristic of his mother, and it cannot be classed among the state-ments which are agreed to in a half-hearted sort of way as not being wrong or as half-true. His mother really must have done particularly fine work.

In another case he told a lady student that her father

generally pushed his glasses up on to his forehead when speaking to anyone, and looked at the person from under them. Whereupon she said that it was quite a characteristic mannerism of her father's.

He told a doctor in the middle of a description of his father that his father had one eye smaller than the other.

He gave a lady from Central Germany a description of her father's grave, with some unusual characteristics. She denied the characteristics, but had to concede that they were correct later on.

Correct statements of this kind in cases where he could not have a chance knowledge of what he described cannot be put down to accident or to guesswork.

(c) **Discussion of the Results**

We will begin by considering the experiments on cryptoscopy. I carried out the experiments purposely in as simple and uniform a manner as possible at the risk of being blamed for their monotony. But it seemed advisable to do so till the existence of cryptoscopy is proved beyond doubt, as it made the evidence obtained more decisive. I did so purposely ; there would have been no difficulty in trying to cause the medium to solve more difficult problems, in looking for changes of meaning (or causing them by suggestion), etc.

It is generally required, and justly so, of decisive experiments on clairvoyance (from which the possibility of telepathy is excluded) that nobody should know what the object under consideration is. I think I have fulfilled this requirement to a large extent. I have not performed any experiments on cryptoscopy where the object was known, with the exception of the last experiment of some of the series with Re, where the slips were all used up ; in all cases but one the slips were written by more than one person or I had written more slips than I actually used ; I could have told the contents of the slip of the 27th experiment if I had been asked, but as a matter of fact, I was attending to the experiment so closely that I did not recall the contents of the slip consciously to mind. It is well to remember that the arrangement of the experiments was such that I had not known and had forgotten the contents of the slips, so that an objection to that effect is unfounded. I could not know the contents of the slip under consideration subconsciously,[1] as I did not know which of my slips he had in his hand. This all the more so as I generally picked the slips out of a larger number I kept in my writing table. As I did not know the contents of the single slips, telepathy can only be taken as an explanation if we suppose that I guessed aright the contents of the slip under consideration every time the answer was given correctly, which itself would have to be explained. For instance, in the second experiment on clairvoyance with Miss von B. (7), I should have to have known not only the contents of three hundred postcards, the position of the different words on them, and the shape of the different letters as well; but even if my conscious mind were gifted in this wonderful way, it would remain to be explained why I should not have communicated the contents of any other card, unless I knew by clairvoyance which it was myself. We cannot eliminate the fact of clairvoyance, so let us look for it in the right place, that is, with Miss von B., and not with me.

Experiments like No. 26 also speak against telepathy. Re read "Brand", then "Braut", "Brett", "Brot", although I did not know what was on the slip to begin with. Naturally enough, I noticed what was on the slip as the experiment went on, but although I knew the contents then, and was thinking of it, Re did not get them right; nor could he get any further, and he had to give up the experiment.

[1] I tried a few experiments on telepathy with Re, but they were all unsuccessful; this is another argument against telepathy as the sole cause or agent in these experiments. This objection is not of a decisive nature (see p. 168).

EXPERIMENTS

We might suspect that telepathy played a part in the 22nd experiment, as it was the last of my slips; but it was not this one Re read; it was the last one of R.'s which was lying on the table. Now R. might have been thinking of the slips, and so communicated the wrong one by mistake; a possibility which cannot be denied in this experiment: but it is a clumsy, complicated explanation, quite unnecessarily so, and it leaves part of the course of the experiment unexplained. So I feel justified in rejecting it. Let us say that this case might be described as suspect, so as to have done with it once for all. Re might have read the slip with the number " 666 " secretly, although he was being closely watched, and nothing led us to believe that he had done so. But a clever conjurer who was not found out under these test conditions could hardly be expected to forget the text of a slip he had read, and then to give that of a wrong one. The simplest explanation in this case is that he was influenced by another slip which he visualized although it was not in his hand. It is not in the nature of clairvoyance to require actual bodily contact with an object in order to be able to perceive it.

The only experiments in which Re was given slips written by persons who were absent were Nos. 69 and 70. The negative results obtained in both cases are no argument for telepathy as against clairvoyance, as Re had practically lost his psychic faculties. So I think we can accept this first point, that the subconscious and telepathy played no part, as proved.

It is rather amusing to see that, when all normal possibilities have failed, people are ready to explain clairvoyance by telepathy, which they had rejected as non-existent but a short time ago, and to accept this rather than accept the simple new fact of clairvoyance *ad hoc*.

The second question we have to deal with is whether or not the medium was really able to read what was written in any normal way. First of all we must consider the possibility of reading letters and slips without opening them. The post cards read by Miss von B. were wrapped up in a piece of black paper, sufficiently large—more than twice the size of the card—so that all the edges were well covered by the paper when it was folded. If we assume that the card was read by transparency we assume that the light (of one candle!) penetrated the two thicknesses of the white envelope, two thicknesses of violet lining, and four thicknesses of opaque black paper, and the post card itself. This is expecting rather much of the light of one candle. It is easy to calculate how many layers the light would have had to penetrate if the card were to be read in this way. I think we can reject both these as possible explanations. It would not be possible to read the slip by the sense of touch through so many thicknesses of paper, especially considering that the writing was in ink. Besides, cotton wool in a small box was very well described in the presence of two witnesses.

Re's method is much the same as that of the clairvoyant Kahn, of whom Schottelius speaks (*Journ. f. Psychol. u. Neurol.*, 1913, vol. 20). Both used small slips folded several times. But Re did not mind how many persons were present, he took the slips in his hand ; both these things Kahn did not do. He does not insist on any act which might distract the attention, like the clairvoyant Reese,[1] so that one can stand quite near him and watch him all the time. As Henning (*Journ. f. Psychol. u. Neurol.*, vol 21) criticized the experiments of Schottelius in great detail, and those with Re are very similar, I must consider them in detail. He maintained that he himself and the people he experimented with could obtain the same results as this type of clairvoyant. I cannot pretend to be able to do the same, although my sight is of more than

[1] Doubts have been raised as to Reese's clairvoyance, but v. Schrenck-Notzing, Maxwell, and Carrington came to the conclusion it was genuine (*Annales*, 1913, vol. 32).

normal keenness, neither has anyone present at the experiments ever thought he could do so under these test conditions.

Henning states that it is possible to read the contents of slips written in pencil by the impression left on the pad. Experiment showed me that this was only possible when thin paper was used and the writer had a heavy hand, but I think that this would hardly be a source of error, as even the most simple and uncritical of experimenters would suspect something if the medium were to investigate the writing pad. I eliminated this possibility in my experiments. In no case was the medium able to see the writing pad ; it was either left in a room the medium did not go into, or it was locked up in a writing table, previous to his entering the room, or else the slips were written on the cover of a pocketbook, which was immediately pocketed. The same may be said of Henning's objection to slips written in ink. He said that the print on the blotting pad could be read; this possibility was also obviated. I only used one such slip (Experiment No. 34).

Henning goes on to say that it is possible for the medium to read the writing by following it with his fingers on the back of the slip as if it were Braille type. I wrote my slips with a very soft pencil, to obviate this possible source of error ; then I smoothed the back of the paper with my thumb nail. In the cases when I wrote only one word or a figure I took care that the written part should not be on the outer layers of the folded slip. Later on I took care that it should be in the middle of the slip, so that it had three thicknesses of paper on the one side and four on the other. I can see only a vain attempt to save " psychology as a science " in the statement of Henning's that the clairvoyant may be able to read the slip with the skin of his forehead. But I am ready to concede this point if Henning is able to read them with his. This does not affect my experiments at all, as Re only very rarely held slips to his forehead ; he did this only when he was in great difficulties, and in a great many of these cases he was not able to read them at all.

I think it most improbable from all my observations (and my attention was concentrated on this point) that the slips should have been unfolded. It is an experiment worth trying, to unfold a slip with one hand, and try to read it, in such a way that persons standing by your side and watching you all the time, never see you do it. It is too much for my credulity to think that this is possible. Even Henning does not pretend that it is possible to unfold a slip completely unobserved even when the observations are being done by the typically simple-minded and credulous observer he has in his mind's eye. He says it might be possible to peep into the slightly opened slip as into an uncut book. I have mentioned previously that I folded my slips with the writing quite in the middle, so that it would be impossible to read them in this way, hence this objection cannot logically be brought up against my experiments.

It must be remembered that Re never tried to divert our attention in any way, and actually would never have succeeded in doing so. *A large number of the experiments were performed in such a way that he held the slip in his left hand with outstretched arm and head turned away so that he looked in the other direction. He remained quite immovable till the answer came.* I was standing or sitting quite close to him, watching him all the time.

The solution of the problem by exchanging the slips *was not possible* in most experiments, as the right number of slips was always in my hands at the end of each series.

It might be suggested that in the cases when I did not write the slips myself, there might have been connivance between Re and the writer. I have known **Mr. R.** for years as a most trustworthy man, and feel quite justified in affirming his reliability. The lady who wrote the slip for the 50th experiment ("Julius") I have known for years as entirely reliable ; she met Re for the first time that evening. She was sitting on a chair twelve feet from Re when he came into the room, and they did not have a chance of coming near to one another. So it is quite impossible that they should have got into communication with one another, and that she should have made a dot on the outside of the slip she gave me for him. But I wrote by far the greater part of the slips myself, and allowed no one a chance of seeing them, so that even if there had been fraud in the above two cases (which seems quite out of the question), it would only explain a small part of the results. This makes the above assumption still more improbable, in fact quite ridiculous.

Collusion with another person present, a scheme often used by conjurers, was not possible either, as I wrote the slips, locked them up in my writing table, and did not take them out until just before the actual experiments. Again, he would not have been able to take them out of my pocket, unfold them, read them, put them back again, and then give them out in the order in which I took them out of my pocket. I do not want to waste time enumerating all the other conjurer's tricks which might have been possible, or rather impossible, under these very strict test conditions ; I can only say that it was quite impossible for anyone conniving with Re to get hold of the slips, and that Re had them at his disposal only for the few moments he took in visualizing them when he held them between thumb and index or in the hollow of his hand, under very close observation, and without making any visible attempts to divert our attention.

So it would be unreasonable to say that there must be a conjuring trick concerned, especially as conjurers are wont to prescribe the conditions and do not work under test conditions of this kind. The conditions can be made simple and open in experiments of this sort. It was my endeavour to take into account all the precautions and objections hitherto suggested, and not only did I fail to detect any fraud (that would mean little), but neither I nor any of my co-workers ever had the faintest impression that there might be a trick of any sort in any part of the experiments. The course of the experiments is so clear and natural and so little suspect, that it would seem quite as logical to suspect that someone who was sitting there talking to me should be committing a murder that very moment.

I am well acquainted with the unreliability of the statements of witnesses, of the psychology of observation, and I think it will be obvious that I went to work very critically myself. We should have to reject all human evidence if we wanted to suspect all these statements.

It is worth calling to mind that there are certain psychic faculties in the animal kingdom—*the instincts* —which are generally recognized, and which we cannot explain at all with our present knowledge of psychology. I particularly want to mention the workings of the instinct of the *Youkka Moth* and the *Sitaris Grub,* which seem to call for clairvoyance in time—prevision— to explain them. To have recourse to such terms as " Inherited habits " or " Mechanized acts of the intellect ", etc., in explanation of these things is to use idle verbiage, much too general to provide us with a true explanation ; it could only deceive the un-critical observer as to our ignorance of the mode of action of instinct or perhaps delude the dogmatist into thinking that there are no gaps or vaguenesses in his systems. The zoologist or psychologist does sometimes speak of " the instinctive acts due to clair-voyance ", using the expression purely as a simile. The collective activity of bees, ants, etc., towards a common goal often does not seem to depend on any kind of language as a mode of inter-communication ;

perhaps we are in the presence of something comparable with or allied to telepathy. Why should we refuse to have anything to do with similar phenomena when we come across them in human beings, because they are but rare and fleeting ; should we not, *instead of expressing surprise*, be prepared rather to find these rudimentary cases of " acts due to clairvoyance " ?[1] Do not the numerous cases of telepathy, clairvoyance, second sight, etc., which keep on reaching our ears, support the existence of such things ? They surely cannot be dismissed with a wave of the hand, even if critics find the great number of these stories suspicious, instead of considering their mere scarcity suspicious, as most people do. You will hardly like to consider these spontaneous cases as the sole proofs of telepathy or clairvoyance, but they can be taken as very good corroborative evidence of such faculties.

As mentioned previously, Re told me himself that he used often to produce " clairvoyance " by a trick. This certainly looks very suspicious, and certainly so it is to a certain extent ; but it is really going too far to refuse to have anything to do with my experiments on these grounds. Paradoxical as it may seem, we can even go so far as to say that it actually speaks for the genuineness of the powers he showed under strict control. Why should he tell me this if he were afraid of suspicion, as he only ran the risk of making us more suspicious by doing so, and of causing us to make the experimental conditions even more rigid, which must be disagreeable to every conjurer ? It would have been rather a rash speculation on Re's part if he had hoped to increase my belief in him by this open statement, and to make me less suspicious. He certainly did not succeed. He showed me tricks several times, and explained them to me.

[1] See my paper in *Psychische Studien*, 1919, Nos. 6 and 7, on " Instinct and Clairvoyance ".

The fact that Re failed completely in the second period of our experiments, when the conditions were no stricter than in the first, if anything less so (in the 69th and 70th experiments I was alone with him so that he had a much better chance of diverting my attention, and thus a better possibility of ascertaining the contents of the slip), rather goes to prove the genuineness of his powers. It is well known that the faculty of clairvoyance is apt to vary or even to cease altogether, and I think that this is the true explanation of the above phenomenon ; it is unusual to forget a trick or to lose the faculty of performing it unless it requires a very difficult technique ; but this is improbable, else why should he not have failed more often in the first series of experiments if that had been the case ? It will be remembered that he had very few failures in the first series. So I think that we can put it down to chance that the only slip correctly seen in the second series was not gummed.

The experiments recorded show that I did not write down the most obvious things on the slips, such as personal associations, though even these allow plenty of chance for variation, and it would really have been extraordinarily lucky if he had got all these right. I want to mention particularly that Mr. R.'s name is not Sebald, and that I was not born in Athens. Those are among the chief objections mentioned by Henning ; it will be seen that I have taken them all into account. There is one point, however, in which I did not let myself be guided by these objections. Henning proposes that one person should write the slip, another should bring it to the person who hands it to the clairvoyant in the experiment, so that no one present should have any knowledge of what is on the slip ; in a great many cases the slips were written by me or by one of the others present. But no one knew the contents of the slip under consideration in my experiments as they were mixed. Hence, this possible source of error could not have played a part in the experiments with post cards with Miss von B.

Among the experiments which might be open to question I want to mention No. 5 and No. 6 with Miss von B. ; had she found out the contents by some fraudulent means during my absence ? It would not have been possible to make the envelope transparent in so short a time by wetting it with alcohol ; besides, the room or the envelope would have smelt of it, traces of its action would have been left on the envelope or on the seals, and I should certainly have noticed something when inspecting the envelope before opening it. Besides black and violet do not become transparent when treated in this way, as a few trials showed me ; they lose some of their colour and dye the neighbouring objects, so that I should most certainly have seen any attempts to treat the envelopes in this way. I think this argument is sufficient to allow us to reject this possibility.

So—unless we accept real clairvoyance—Miss von B. must have opened the gummed envelope which had five seals, read it, and reclosed it in such a way that I could detect absolutely no traces of this in the space of five minutes, regardless of the fact that I looked into the room several times. This is the only remaining possibility I can think of, and it seems quite pre-posterous to imagine that she performed such a feat in so short a time. I think we can say that it was a technical impossibility, and that to maintain this suggestion as a fact would be to expect too much of the medium's technical skill and of our powers of belief—a belief which would be suspiciously like the " credo, quia absurdum est "—. Braid, the discoverer of hypnotism, once said, " Absolute scepticism is as much the child of intellectual limitation as absolute credulity." I think that the man who doubts the evidence of these experiments might come under the former category. We must remember that Miss von B.

had neither my violet sealing-wax, my seal, nor any of these envelopes at her disposal. If she had used the same envelope we should certainly have detected traces of her opening it. All this can be regarded as quite impossible, especially as I kept peeping in secretly. The sceptic will say that when something so incredible as clairvoyance is in question, something which upsets all our theories, the man who claims the existence of such a thing must prove it. This may be all right as a matter of fact, but it does not mean that the sceptic is justified in bringing up the most absurd possibilities against it. He is not justified in thinking that he can maintain anything he likes, and that it is the duty of others to disprove all of these often underground speculations. Such a mode of action may be all right in the law courts but happily in science we are not dealing with a mass of dead and formal paragraphs in which we are wound up as in a net, which tends to choke all good, common-sense thinking. Here, we must consider the actual facts quite objectively, and so the wilder and more improbable the assertions of the opponents of new facts, the better it is for those who are trying to gain recognition for them, and I maintain that the statement claiming that the letter was opened is so improbable that the other alternative gains a very high degree of probability by such an assertion in the face of the evidence ; in fact we may take it as proved. Wasielewski's book, in which all his experiments with Miss von B. are recorded, appeared since the publication of this book, and describes a whole series of experiments in which the medium was being watched all the time—-this, by the way, was before my experiments with Miss von B.

At any rate, the right to ignore this whole mass of observations cannot be justly claimed as it has been up to now, in the face of such evidence ; they can say that " it is worth considering ", " probable ", or even " very probable ". How many of the generally accepted theories of natural science rest on really sound proofs ? Often the actual proof has not yet been given or may be impossible to give. This is true, for instance, of the Theory of the Ether, the Darwinian Theory, and the Atomic Theory. The latter has been doubted of late by no less a scientist than Ostwald, although it had been accepted definitely for a long time, and now it seems as firmly established as ever. The Darwinian Theory was once generally accepted, and has now been abandoned by many ; yet at one time it was defended with fanaticism. This should make scientists more tolerant and lead them to recognize that there are other alternatives than merely denying, ignoring, or accepting a thing.

It seems to me that if we consider all the pros and cons in this series of experiments, it is not the probability of real clairvoyance that we are considering but the proof of its actual existence, unless we still maintain that a letter sealed five times could be opened and closed in such a way as not to show a single trace of the fact under my supervision. To this evidence we must add the positive experiments with Re and the experiment with the box containing cotton wool, which was done in the continuous presence of two people besides myself.

Chance cannot be invoked as an explanation of these facts, as I mentioned previously, when discussing Henning's objections (p. 150) ; it would be too fantastic a chance. Is it within the range of probability that the clairvoyant should guess right the answers of the four slips given him in one sitting, as was the case in the experiments Nos. 26–30, and that he should guess that the words " Brot ", " Barbara ", " Agathe ", and the number " 21244 " were on these slips ? Things like this must be emphasized when we see how the experiments of other investigators have been treated. Hopp writes as follows (p. 73) about Richet's experiments with drawings : " Now we come to the experiments with drawings. Here the theory of probabilities is not applicable. It is impossible to give in numbers the probability of the correct reproduction of an imaginary picture drawn for the purpose of reproduction, as the number of possible drawings is incalculable. *Therefore these experiments have no decisive value whatsoever* according to my mind, although the last experiment described is most striking." It is true that there is a certain vague analogy which may crop up by chance in drawings, and which should not mislead the critical observer ; there is something angular, triangular, rectangular, or circular in most drawings. But to say that these experiments can have " no evidential value " whatever, because the theory of probabilities is not applicable to them, is surely a caricature of the much-needed mathematical accuracy in science. This kind of scepticism has nothing in common, except the name, with the justified methodical scepticism of science, and is really quite as unmethodical as utter lack of criticism. In many of my experiments it is not possible to calculate the probabilities of finding a word correctly, still less of seeing several words in their correct places on a post card, and writing them with several of their characteristics. Does Hopp wish to maintain that these experiments " have no evidential value whatever ", because of that ?

I myself have tried to satisfy the demands of such sharp critics : unfortunately, for several reasons, I was prevented from making as long and as regular a series of experiments as I should have liked to make. Re knew that I had written five figures of three digits each in experiments 16 to 24. As the last was not used there remain four slips, three of which were read correctly ; the probability of succeeding in doing that was 1 : 7,290,000. Now the experiment was somewhat complicated by the fact that R. had also provided five slips, which reduces the probability to less than half of the above. At any rate, this is the hint of a mathematical treatment of the question, and it does not speak in favour of the results being due to chance. The fact that Hopp brings up the impossibility of mathematical treatment against Kotik and Wasielewski, shows what weight he lays upon it. I want to discuss the experiments on psychoscopy separately, as they require different treatment owing to their characteristic peculiarities. It seems to me that even the most decided sceptic should be somewhat startled by such results and have cause to think. As already mentioned they are often vague, and the exact calculation of the probabilities is not possible, but I fancy that they are not without any evidential value all the same. As I have maintained above, the results should be weighed and not simply expressed in numbers. The statement that an object comes from an unmarried man or woman might have a probability of, say, 20 per cent. More descriptive statements which apply to fewer people would have to be valued with a lower coefficient of probability ; a characteristic statement which is outside all probability has more value than a number of negative statements. The coincidence of a number of correct statements gives us the greatest probability that they are not due to chance. So that it can frankly be said that, although the probabilities cannot be calculated, *the statements that an object was presented by an elderly gentleman to a thin young man, and is brought into connexion with a silk suit, a watering-place on the Baltic, and a 'cello,* cannot be put down to chance. Or is it not most improbable that *a rosary should have been described, as far as its outside form is concerned, out of the multitude of possible things which might have been taken, and, as in experiment No. 82, the impressions connected with the object should have been described beyond possible confusion ; that the right verses should have been so characteristically rendered out of all the possible verses which might have been chosen, or that Miss von B. should have described a wedding on an estate in an unmistakable manner* (No. 79); *although these things cannot be treated mathematically by the calculation of probabilities?* (see also No. 150). Is it not a strange " coincidence " that *a child should appear* (No. 115) *and be correctly described doing an action connected with the object* the very first time the object came from a child (see also No. 173) ; *that a weapon from the stone age should be characterized as such ; that the figure and the frame on the hundred rouble note should be described?* I have only just alluded to a very few of the experiments so as to put them in their true light, and did not mean to refer to all the successful ones. It might be well to refer to Nos. 96, 109, 112, 118, 119, 126, 128, 139, 142, 145.

Supposing a man sitting in a room hears 100 shots fired at some distance from the house ; some of the shots whirr past the house and he sees that it has been struck 30 times ; he will surely not conclude that someone was potting about aimlessly with his gun but that he was shooting at the house, and his conclusion will be justified as, otherwise, one shot at most would have struck the house. In our experiments we must not consider the shots which flew past the house but those that struck it, which are much more numerous than we should be led to expect by working out the probabilities. In other words, if such a coincidence is found in a series of experiments, the methodical observer will say it is a curious coincidence, but if they are as numerous as above, he will have to look for some other factor than chance ; now, as guesswork and tricks are excluded by the arrangement of the experiments, he will have to look for some quite different cause (*vide infra*). This is a step which may be very difficult to thinkers who have got into a groove, whose views all run in a direction which is hardly or not at all compatible with these facts ; but this step will have to be taken, just as Schopenhauer had to face these facts towards the end of his life. He dealt with them

EXPERIMENTS

positively in a most capable manner, in a way which
often contradicted his earlier statements down to their
very fundamentals.

A world in which chance coincidences were as frequent
as is suggested would be comparable with the world
of fairy tales and can be rejected straight away as
unreal. I, for one, am not going to venture into such a
world ; the occult world seems to me to be a world of
law and order compared to this one, although it is
weird at times.

It is usual in scientific research to test a given factor
by eliminating it in parallel series of experiments, so
that the way to prove the normal origin of such facts
would be to repeat these experiments under the same
conditions with a series of persons who are not mediums.
I have done this in a number of cases and have found
that chance could not produce such results. It was
very rarely that statements were made which could be
brought into relation with the object in any way. And
these statements were of a very general nature, for
instance : " Tender memories are associated with the
object," etc. We were able to observe among other
things that objects, even if they are not wrapped up
in any way, can lead to a great variety of different
statements, so that it is very difficult to say correct
things about them ; in fact is is often misleading to
know the object ; general statements about its use and
associations are often wrong, as the objects are generally
chosen because they have a *history*.

I have suggested to my opponents that they should
try such experiments. Strange to say, my suggestion
fell on deaf ears, and yet such experiments are perfectly
easy to do. Are they afraid that their results might
help to prove the correctness of my statements ? It is
no use to say that they have not suitable subjects ;
anyone who does not possess such inhibitions that he
cannot say what comes into his mind can act as a
subject. If the critics think they must have persons

with the imaginative power of a Mr. H. they will find that the statements go further afield, as persons of that type have a wider " angle of divergence " in their statements, owing to their imagination.

It may be said, and it has been said, that H. has complexes which come up more frequently. That is possible (e.g. a middle-aged lady, etc.), but even if such complexes were much more frequent than they actually are, they do not cover the important points. Either the complex is of a general nature, and the observer will not lay much stress on those data, or the complex will have exact and characteristic details which are most unlikely to fit the subject ; if it does happen to fit it once in a while it will do so very rarely indeed, as we can see by working out the probabilities, so rarely that it would make no practical difference in the final result of the series. For instance, the " War-complex ", which is not at all far-fetched and which often appears when we try experiments with normal, non-sensitive persons, does not appear very often with H., and then mostly when the object is really connected with war (Nos. 82, 96, 142).

A critic thinks that the sense of smell may have played a part in the experiments. He bases his statements on the fact that certain insects can find their mates at a distance of several miles by the sense of smell. As in that case the minutest traces of a thing would be sufficient to cause a sense-perception, he says it might be the case here, too, e.g. in No. 83, a few molecules of sea air might have remained attached to the object and might have called forth a vision of, or statements about, the sea, by association with the smell of seaweed. This does not seem very probable to me, but this probability decreases immensely when we find that this button was kept in an old cigar box, as long as I can remember it, and this box in a cupboard with chemicals such as iodoform and lysol, a smell which still clings to that cupboard after all these years. One would expect these strong smells to have obscured the smell of seaweed, so that if smell really did play a part we should have been drawn into medical surroundings instead.

As already mentioned, all the persons present during the experiments, including the members of the Medical Commission, were of the opinion that fraud was impossible under these conditions, and that any voluntary or involuntary exchange of signals was out of the question in the experiments, where no one present knew what the object was ; the only remaining alternatives were chance of supernormal faculty of some kind. So that the reader has all the data required to be able to form an opinion on the subject, for any doubts which might arise (such as those of fraud in séances for physical phenomena) are eliminated by the simple and clear order of experimentation and the judgment of so many people. They just have to consider the records and to form their judgment.

I resist the temptation of giving a false impression of accuracy by splitting the data of the experiments into their different components, and then calculating how many of them are right, indifferent, or wrong. This pseudo-exactitude would give us quite a wrong picture of the experiments, and that not always to their *disadvantage*. It is quite possible that the percentage of correct statements would be very high in an experiment which we should not think of putting among the best, as the statements might be of an indifferent nature. These experiments cannot be adequately treated by the theory of probabilities as it is not the number of correct statements which gives them their true value but the quality of these statements ; they must be, as it were, weighed. A really very characteristic statement may outweigh a number of erroneous or general statements.

Of course, there are a number of events which are more or less generally applicable to some objects.

For instance, most tie-pins go for a railway journey now and again ; that is why I have not taken a number of correct statements of this type into account in my commentaries. But in a great many cases we find ourselves face to face with coincidences which refer to such special things that the above observation can hardly account for them. In some experiments there is not a single statement which can be proved to be accurate, and incorrect or false statements are often mixed up with them, but this does not detract from the value of the correct statements. Suppose an angler to come back often from fishing without any fish, that does not make the fish he brings back any less real.

I once wanted to see what chance would do, so I took the objects and the results of a series of 11 experiments I had before me and drew lots to see how they would come together. This was the result :

Object.	*Result.*
Silver dish (79)	Coin (96)
Letter scales (80)	Watch glass (81)
Watch glass (81)	Tie-pin (92)
Mirror (82)	Poem (97)
Button (83)	Button (83)
Rosary (89)	Mirror (82)
Tie-pin (92)	Silver dish (79)
Vase (95)	Letter scales (80)
Coin (96)	Vase (95)
Poem (97)	Entrance card (100)
Entrance card (100)	Rosary (89)

If we compare this with the text we shall not, I think, find many chance coincidences ; as far as I can see, the number of correct statements would not increase if we began investigations on the basis of the above result. It is not unnatural that there should be one coincidence in such a small number of cases, and yet this does not make an appreciable difference in the main question before us.

EXPERIMENTS

I am not going into the mathematical aspects of the theory of probabilities, for two reasons; first, I am no mathematician, and secondly, it is not applicable numerically to these experiments. I only want to make a few remarks. As far as I know, the mathematician needs long series of results, and this is necessary beyond doubt in cases where you are not dealing with simple problems, say, with the figures between 1 and 10, or with playing cards (1 : 52). In our experiments, where the number of possibilities is so great, a single correct statement will have a very much lower coefficient of probability, and therefore a much higher value ; now, if there are several correct statements in one such experiment, these coefficients sink very rapidly, and with them the possibility of putting the result down to chance, and we soon reach coefficients such as are generally found in other scientific investigations. Strictly speaking, we are dealing with probabilities all the time in scientific investigations, in so far as we are investigating inductively discovered data.

Therefore, supernormal perceptions must play a part in these experiments ; there are two which suggest themselves at once, clairvoyance and telepathy. The latter possibility cannot be excluded in the experiments where anyone knew what the object of the particular experiment was ; but the results of these experiments were so very similar to those of the experiments in which no one present knew the object that it is certainly simpler to suppose that clairvoyance was the agency at work in both kinds.

There are other points in favour of putting the results down to clairvoyance. As already mentioned, I tried experiments in telepathy several times with H., in which Gruber or I were the agents. We tried these experiments both when H. was in his normal condition and when he was in trance, but we never obtained results which were better than what you might expect from chance. This result, of course, only applies to telepathy from the conscious mind. This type of experiment can afford no clue whatever about telepathy from the unconscious. But we must consider one thing. H. often gives information which has nothing to do with the object in hand as far as we can tell ; a glance at the records will show this at once. We have never noticed that these statements were connected in any way with things which were occupying our minds, or that they were connected with things we knew, and which would have been characteristic of any one of us. So, if we were to ascribe the statements of H., in the cases in which we knew the object, to telepathy from the subconscious (which would be possible, for it can hardly be supposed that our total knowledge of an object should be in our minds all the time), we shall have to explain why those particular mental data and not others were transmitted, and this, as we saw, was not the case. These facts do not tend to make us ascribe our results to telepathy whether it come from the conscious or the subconscious mind.

Now, it is a remarkable fact that a whole series of experiments done in the autumn of 1920, in which the objects were known, gave particularly good results (Nos. 139–150). The data given not only referred to the history of the object, but also to its form and consistency. Things like that happened also in experiments in which the object was not known ; for instance, in experiment No. 119 when the bronze medal was described, and then H. was in very good condition ; his health had improved and financial difficulties which had been weighing upon him had come to an end. But the available material does not seem sufficient to decide the question.

The scope of telepathy has been very much extended by some investigators ; they maintain that all statements made by the seer about anything that anyone on earth knows are due to telepathy. Professor

Oesterreich tried to show that all the facts given by clairvoyants, especially those of psychoscopy, were all due to telepathy. He says that mediums of this type are in telepathic relation with almost everybody in the world, and so have access by telepathy to almost everything that other people experience, or have stored up anywhere in their memories.

He even maintains that the data of events long past are also due to telepathy, as all persons of a mediumistic nature would be in unconscious telepathic rapport and so anything that anybody had ever known would be passed on from generation to generation. This theory is most interesting, but is it capable of explaining all the facts ? It does not say how the medium gets on the track of the object ; and we must not forget that vision into the past is intimately connected with the parallel phenomenon, vision into the future, which from its very nature cannot be accounted for by telepathy as above defined. This makes us rather sceptical about this explanation of vision in the past. Oesterreich calls this faculty " Paramnesia ".

But there are other ways in which the results of our experiments in psychoscopy seem to speak against this theory ; as we have seen, we cannot say that the experiments in which the object was known gave us better results than the others, even if we take into account all the modifying conditions. If we say that the seer should be able to read the minds of all men, then it is not clear why he does not try to do so at first with those who are present, which should not have been difficult, as he knew who had chosen the object in a great many cases, even when several people were present.

It might be objected that I have called a number of experiments positive in which chance might have played a part. But it seems to me that it would certainly be a *petitio principii* to call these cases positive if there were no other strikingly positive statements. As H. makes a number of most strikingly characteristic statements, in which chance cannot play a part, I feel quite justified in assuming that the same supernormal faculty played a part in these, and that I need not expect " chance " to do all this. This type of experiment on clairvoyance has the advantage that it is not open to the accusation of being due to tricks, for even the cleverest conjurer cannot recognize things which are not present unless he is a clairvoyant as well. If we take enough precautions, there is no doubt that such experiments in psychoscopy may produce most valuable material. *These experiments alone would suffice to prove the existence of clairvoyance. So we must recognize that such different series of experiments performed with different mediums are a very much more conclusive proof.* Trickery, chance, and guesswork, the favourite loopholes of the sceptic, are useless against such evidence ; we cannot but accept the fact of clairvoyance.

So there is nothing left but to face the view that there are extrasensuous, supernormal ways of receiving knowledge of things, and become acquainted with this abnormality. You cannot do justice to the problem by ignoring it, denying it, or using such excuses as trickery, chance, or guesswork. We must master those facts regardless of whether they are explicable by the " scientific views " held in 1921. Whether they are explicable or not cannot be a criterion as to whether facts should be accepted or rejected.

It is particularly disturbing that a person with the necessary faculties should be able to visualize scenes, and to follow the affective tone of happenings which occurred years, even tens of years, ago, simply by being in the presence of an object connected with them. The supernormal influences were not so strong with H. as they were with Miss von B., and his imagination was very much more active, so that they were easily swamped by his stream of normal thought, and what made things more difficult still, he had no judgment as to whether or not a statement was correct. As a consequence disturbing factors of any kind (e.g. suggestion, etc.) have a strong effect on H. and tend to repress the supernormal influences.

Let us next inquire, by considering the experiments with post cards and slips, if we can find out how this knowledge is obtained. I will begin by saying at once that the result is negative, but we shall come across a few interesting facts all the same. We will consider the post cards first. It might be supposed that the position of the words might have some influence on their being read. We might think that the beginnings and endings of the lines were read more easily in the first post card (No. 6 : Karte, gut, schaft, verstreut), but this is a vague surmise which is rendered still more unlikely by the second post card (No. 7). Here, except for the beginning and the end of the text ("Endlich kann" and "Lina Luder"), we have a word in the middle of a line (jetzt) and the end of a line (Mein Vater). In fact, we may say that if we consider the analogy with ordinary reading, we should expect more beginnings and endings to have been read. It seems that, apart from the beginning and the end, the words read were strewn promiscuously all over the card. We cannot pretend either that particularly conspicuous words were read; neither "Jahr" nor "jetzt" strike the eye when first looking at the card. The recognition of the syllable "schaft" out of the middle of the word "landschaftlich" is very strange ; the syllable as it was seen made no sense. The word "verstreut" which was read without reference to the context, as the last thing on that side of the card, is not easy to read by normal sight, except in context. Whereas in many cases the meaning was felt intuitively as already mentioned, here it seems to have been a case of pure visual perception, and yet, as far as we know, the picture-forming part of the eye does not have anything to do with the process.

The next thing worth mentioning is that the letters often bear a strong resemblance to the originals, or at any rate belong to the same type. The "F" in "Frau" (Figs. 3, 4) belongs to quite a different type from the "F" in "Familie" (Figs. 6*a*, 7*a*), yet in both cases Miss von B. kept to the type of the original, although she did not reproduce it exactly. There are other similarities which cannot be put down to chance, e.g. the "z" in "jetzt" is drawn towards the "t" in quite a characteristic way; the "V" in "Vater" has twice the same transition to the "a"; the "L" in "Luder" seems to be an exact copy of the original, the "d" goes straight into the "l" at the top on the word "endlich", etc. However, we must not forget that there are great differences sometimes, as for instance the "K" in "Karte", and the "M" in "Mein₄". I have the impression that the copying was done practically unconsciously, so that it is no wonder that some letters turned out to be very different; Miss von B. had not been told to copy the writing exactly. We do sometimes happen to make use of an unusual type of letter when we are copying something, especially when we are dreaming. We can take it for granted that the consciousness is somewhat repressed, or at any rate narrowed down in practising clairvoyance, even in the case of waking clairvoyance; this is confirmed by the seers being so influenced by the visualized writing. (See Wasielewski's book on Miss von B.: *Telepathie und Hellsehen.*)

I often asked Re to write words just as he saw them. The resemblance to the original writing is obvious (No. 20 Eberhard, No. 22 München, Figs. 8, 9, 10, and 11), but he, too, sometimes makes mistakes, for instance he dotted a ɪ, or used a different type of letter altogether (No. 32, mandoline). The intentional mistake, and the form of the letter "C" were perfectly recognized in the word Canstatt (No. 43, Figs. 16 and 17). Here also we have a kind of "optical" recognition of the object, which is still more striking in No 38 when he reads the word " panta rei " which is meaningless to him, or tries to draw a few Sanscrit letters in No. 39 (Figs. 14 and 15).

Very curious are the remarks he makes sometimes ; for instance, in No. 26 that it is a quotation, or in No. 28. Oddly enough, he says something which is not included and cannot be derived from the data he gives, e.g. he could not conclude from the word " Brot " (bread) that it was a quotation. This points to the fact that there is another " non-optical " factor beside the above-mentioned optical factor. We find the same thing with Kotik and Chowrin. This is particularly the case with the " thought-laden " paper, and in the psychoscopical experiments it seems as if a fragment of the mind of the person were attached to the object, and as if this were not always connected intimately with the written statement.

We often find slight divergences from the original (e.g. No. 35 Madelene instead of Madalene, No. 42 Zarastro instead of Sarastro). There are but few absolutely incorrect statements in the first period, e.g. " Anna or Unna " instead of " Frommert " (No. 40). Unfortunately I did not go into the matter thoroughly at the time ; if I had done so, possibly I might have found some clue.

So we cannot pretend to have got any nearer to the solution of this dilemma by studying the experiments more closely.

It does not seem to affect the reading of the slip at all whether or not the writing was folded up with the slip, or what was the position of the letters or words to one another, as they lay in the folded slip ; they sometimes lay in superposed layers, so that if they had been read by normal sight on transparent paper only a general medley of superimposed letters would have been seen. This is a strange fact which makes it much more difficult to find an explanation. R. Meyer (*Berl. klin. Wochenschrift*, 1914, p. 1978) took the trouble to try this. He wrote slips such as Schottelius and I had used, traced them on a film and folded it ; nobody was able to read them, not even the clairvoyant with whom Schottelius had experimented. A great many people will have concluded that this jumble of lines could not be read with the human eye, and that the clairvoyant cannot do that either. But this fact cannot be used a priori against the possibility of reading slips by clairvoyance. For instance, one evening at a sitting a number of figures which were written on slips without any overlapping were not read ; the only slip read that evening was the one inscribed with the word " Julius " where the two last letters were folded back over the two middle ones, so that only the first two letters were free (No. 50).

Let us proceed to some general remarks on the psychoscopical experiments, without going into too much detail. The perceptions in these experiments are often of the nature of very vivid optical perceptions, visions, and then H. has often acoustical perceptions, auditions, " they tell him," and these voices have different characteristics ; they are often inner voices, but they are sometimes of the nature of an acoustical hallucination ; they seem to him to come from the outside, to have an objective character, and he tries to fend them off. When not in trance he does not consider them to be really objective. When he judges them, he quite realizes that they do not correspond to any fact outside himself, but that it is only a case of hallucination. So that the auditions have the general character of perceptions, and the visions the more conceptual character of images ; these are so life-like that H. took them to be perceptions till I had explained to him the difference between the two (e.g. Nos. 139 and 157). He describes the apparition of these images as follows.

It seems to him as if he were looking into turbid water, which seems to get clearer gradually, and in which the objects appear, first vaguely, then more clearly. These visions have not the characteristics of reminiscences, and strange to say, H. has no notion whether they are correct or not. Some of the visions which are not connected with the object in any way can be remarkably life-like.

He can make no statements about the psychical phenomena which occur during his trances, as he comes out of trance with amnesia ; but it is possible to arrive at a few conclusions on the subject by watching his behaviour. In No. 109 he behaved as if he were in Dr. R.'s laboratory. He pointed to the chemical apparatus on the table, went to the bookshelf and pointed to the different volumes as he counted them. He sat down again and then came out of trance suddenly. In a negative experiment in which Dr. von Hattingberg was present he got up and pointed to some pictures he seemed to see on the wall and described them ; this time he fell into trance so gradually that Dr. von H., who is a nerve specialist with a wide experience, never noticed the change in his state of consciousness ; I had a sort of feeling that he was not in his normal condition and asked him later on about his getting up and walking about ; it appeared that he knew nothing about it, so he had actually been in trance.

These optical and acoustical impressions in the waking state must be judged quite differently. There were scenes which actually, or very probably, had some connexion with the object at the back of the visual perceptions ; whereas the acoustical perceptions seem—as far as I can see—to be of an unreal or symbolical nature, and do not correspond to anything which actually occurred ; it is " said " to him. They are not sensual—supersensual experiences like the visions ; they are only information which is imparted to him in some other way, clothed in an acoustic garment. He receives these auditions during crypto-scopy as well as during psychoscopy; they call to him " It is a ring ", as well as " Christmas ". He has vivid visions in both the above cases, too.[1]

Besides the two here described modes of percep-tion, he also receives information in a third way, which has no analogy in the physical world. For instance, H. says that he felt the atmosphere of the poem (Stimmung) without having any optical or acoustical perceptions or conceptions to impart this knowledge to him. This same direct knowledge appears in No. 155 (that it is a present, and not an heirloom). I do not wish to say that it really is direct knowledge, and that there are no perceptions at the back of it which did not rise into consciousness or were not remembered.

Most of the information comes as visions and as knowledge, which are in some way connected with the fate of the object or of its owner, these being mostly events which happened to him while in possession of the object. But it seems possible for the clairvoyant to be able to feel his way onward, e.g. the little vase was not yet in the possession of Mrs. T. when she left Genoa ; it was bought in Athens on the return journey ; she did not go to Genoa again.

Let us analyse our results from another point of view. We have statements which are of a cryptoscopic nature in the narrow sense of the word, i.e. the sayings of the seer about things, their properties, etc., sayings which he could have made if he had had the object before him, e.g. the rouble note, the locket, etc. Also, he gives information about scenes which the object has experienced in its life, or, to put it less vividly, scenes from its history. There again he mentions things which are not directly connected with the object, e.g. an experience of the owner of the object

[1] Compare this with my article on the state of consciousness of mediums in *Psychische Studien*, 1921. August.

before it was in his possession (the silver notebook, and the preparation in alcohol in No. 112). Then we have statements which depend on an intuitive knowledge, which are pure thoughts or " consciousnesses " (Bewusstheiten) about things. These can also be divided into two categories corresponding to the two above categories, but there is no parallel to the third. We first have the statements he made about the poems ; he did not read the words but was conscious of, or felt and knew, the general note of the poem ; then statements like that in No. 109, when he said " there is love connected with it ", etc. As above mentioned, this intuitive consciousness of things sometimes appears in the garb of an audition.

It is clear that analysis shows us all sorts of categories of the main phenomenon. We have cryptoscopy, vision into the past, both in space and time, and then the difference between the intuitive and perceptive parts. We may ask ourselves whether all these different phenomena are due to one and the same mental process ; they seem to require the action of several different ones. We shall feel particularly inclined to separate the intuitive phenomena from the perceptive. On the other hand, the fact that these different phenomena appear mixed up without any sequence or order in the statements made by H. speaks very strongly for the fact that they are closely related to one another. There is no indication that one of these groups is peculiar to the experiments in which the object is known, and that it should point to telepathy.

Its origin is still an enigma—especially the intuitive consciousness of things or events ; we can say very little about it. Are there really merely processes which are only in the realm of thought, of purely mental origin, or is there a supersensuous act of perception at the back of them which does not come into consciousness, and the results of which appear as abstract knowledge of things ? We know practically nothing about this ; so it seems to me that we can classify all these phenomena under the heading of clairvoyance, although this abstract " knowing " is not " seeing " ; especially as it is usual to include clairaudience, etc., under the same heading in ordinary conversation, and we speak of a person having this gift of foreknowledge be it intuitive or not—as a " seer ".

We can accept this term as applying to a category of phenomena until our knowledge is sufficient to enable us to coin suitable words in true accordance with these phenomena. But we must remember that the name clairvoyance does not imply any particular explanation of the facts.

As already mentioned, the phenomena of Mr. H. remind us of the processes which take place in dreams ; this is quite natural as in both cases we have psychic processes of the subconscious before us. A typical example of this is the statement that they keep on telling him " Ganges on the Benares " although he knows it is not correct—this is just the sort of thing each of us experiences in his dreams. In dreams we experience all these different dissociations of a personality which is undivided in the daytime, and see two different layers holding two different opinions and disagreeing with one another. These other personalities which he considers as unfriendly often give him information which he refuses to accept, but which sometimes turns out not to be quite wrong, e.g. the mention of the ribbon of the iron cross in No. 96, a statement which is worth further notice. We are led to take into further consideration statements which are not absolutely correct according to the letter of the word, by the manner in which the statements are produced, and sometimes to judge them as positive, for instance the mention of the ribbon of the iron cross, and that of the stars in No. 92. It will be wise to wait till we have collected more material before proceeding to an exact psychological analysis of cases of this type.

EXPERIMENTS

Dr. Schede subsequently sent me the following commentary on the experiments he had witnessed: "The experiments I witnessed with Miss von B., in 1913, have led me to conclude that it was a case of genuine clairvoyance, as trickery and other modes of deception were made impossible by the arrangement of the experiments.

"The only positive experiment which I witnessed with Re was carried out under conditions which rendered fraud impossible."

Dr. Paul Flaskämper writes : "I was able to observe the experiments with the clairvoyant Re very closely (I sat five feet from him), and could watch every movement from his taking the slip which was handed to him, or rather from the writing of the slips to the answer of the clairvoyant. Tricks or fraud were not possible owing to the simple and clear nature of the experiments, which fulfilled all the requirements of accurate scientific work. The successful experiment made an absolutely conclusive impression on me."

Mr. Kuttner, who had made a special study of conjuring and of the possibilities of imitating the results of telepathy and clairvoyance, was present during experiments Nos. 75 to 78. I had asked him to pay particular attention to any sign of attempts at trickery. The experiments were performed in exactly the same way as Nos. 31 to 33, so that Mr. K. could see under what conditions these successful experiments had been performed. So that the judgment of an independent witness who was acquainted with both these branches is valuable, although he did not see any really positive experiments with Re. Mr. K. writes : "I was present at the experiments arranged by Dr. Tischner, and came to the conclusion that Re did not make any use of conjuring tricks. At any rate, none of the usual tricks which are used in ' natural magic ', especially tricks with the hands, seem to have been used, in my opinion. Mr. Re did not show any such technique nor that peculiar neatness of action which is usual with conjurers. So I fancy that there was no fraud in the series of experiments carried on in this way."

Dr. Bormann, an experienced occultist, told me that there could have been no fraud in the experiments he had witnessed. He said that he had never seen such successful and absolutely conclusive experiments.

Professor Gruber writes in the following terms : " Any attempt at fraud on the part of a medium, who worked in full daylight, and under our direct supervision, could have been prevented with perfect ease in the numerous experiments (26) of Dr. Tischner's, with Mr. H. in which I kept the records. It would not have been possible to guess what were the objects (which were tightly packed) by shaking, fingering, hearing, etc. We gave no help in words ; besides, in a great many of the experiments, we did not know what the objects were. Anyone who has witnessed such a large number of positive experiments knows that it is impossible that chance should have played an important part in securing the results. The only factor which remains to account for them is supernormal faculty. As experiments in which the object was known to no living person were positive, I take it that clairvoyance is definitely proved, telepathy being impossible in the circumstances. I should not like to pronounce a final judgment as to how far telepathy was concerned in the experiments in which the object was known. It is quite possible that telepathy did play a part, but even then we cannot account for all the statements made in the experiments unless we concede that clairvoyance played a part in them too."

I consider that this statement, from the member of the medical commission who witnessed so many experiments, commands attention. The man with the best knowledge on the subject should be able to pass the best judgment on the experiments. This is the case in other branches of science. The commission as a whole has not passed a definite judgment on the subject as the experiments have not yet been finished.

SUMMARY

I may now summarize the results of the different classes of experiments. To begin with, there are four positive experiments in telepathy with mediums whose honesty is beyond doubt. The arrangement of the experiments was such that they could not be affected by unconscious whispering, chance, or other sources of error. This allows us to say that *these experiments are proofs of supersensual thought-transference*, as it is only necessary to have a few faultless experiments in science to prove the existence of a phenomenon.

The first two experiments in clairvoyance with Miss von B. were carried out under conditions which excluded any possibility of fraud ; anyone knowing Miss von B. as I have got to know her in the course of time, would reject the idea. But as I got to know her only after our experiments I took all the precautions that should be taken with an unknown medium and watched her with the greatest care. The reader will remember that I observed her through the gap of the door which I had left ajar several times and never saw anything to arouse the slightest suspicion. The third experiment was carried out in such a way that two persons were present during the whole of the experiment ; this experiment was positive also. The success of this experiment supports the evidence derived from the first two experiments with post cards, so that I can *regard the reality of clairvoyance as proved by these three experiments, in which fraud and chance could not have played a part.* For the objection that Miss von B. could have gained a knowledge of the contents by opening the envelopes and closing them in the space of five minutes, without any technical appliances, and without my noticing anything whenever I looked in, cannot be taken seriously.

Then we have the experiments with Re, which were often performed in such a way that I handed him a slip the contents of which were unknown to both of us ; this he took in his hand, and I stood next to him till he had given us the result. Re held this slip to one side and looked in the opposite direction, remaining immovable all the time. He made no attempt to read it, to hold it to his forehead, to put it into the other hand or to do anything else with it from the moment he took it to the end of his answer. The slip was there immovable in the hand with which he had taken it without its being opened to the slightest extent ; on the contrary he generally held it tightly between thumb and index finger. I would again insist that Re never tried to distract our attention in any way. He did not influence the experimental order in any way, and played a purely passive part in most experiments. He stood there, and took the slip I gave him ; then he remained without moving till he had given the answer, when I took the slip out of his hand.

The results of the experiments with Miss von B. are strongly corroborated by the number of positive experiments with Re in which chance and fraud were excluded also. The experimental order was quite different in this series, so if there were a flaw in them we should have to look for it in a different place from the first series. We should have to conclude that there were *two* different sources of error which were misleading us in these two series ; and this reduces the probability of the existence of two such sources.

The large number of psychoscopical experiments also points to the action of some supernormal faculty ; and although telepathy is not excluded in many cases, the number of positive experiments in which the object was unknown is amply sufficient to prove the presence of clairvoyance, as the statements were often much too highly specialized in character to be considered explicable by chance. The large amount of material I have collected in my book *Ludwig Aub* also goes to support this.

The reader should remember that I am not a novice who has waded into these investigations without any previous knowledge of the subject, simply out of curiosity. I have given years of study to occultism. I had had many an unsuccessful experiment and many a case of fraud before I planned and carried out my experiments with Re. I think I know the crucial points of experiments of this type, and I carried them out with the greatest care, so that it would have taken uncommon stupidity and clumsiness for me to have fallen into a trap. I have a very fair knowledge of the psychological and neurological literature on the subject, especially of the objections raised against clairvoyance and telepathy. I had written a critical account of Henning's publication which contained most of the possible and impossible objections against these two faculties (*Psychische Studien*, 1918, Nos. 280–84) before beginning my experiments with Re.

Not one of the persons who witnessed the experiments in my rooms has given voice to the least doubt, and some of them had come to the sittings certain that the whole thing was a fraud. It is symptomatic of this field of research that persons who have been to experiments begin to have doubts *subsequently,* as to the genuineness of the phenomena. But neither I nor any of the small circle of people who were present at the different experiments felt this ; the longer I went on with the experiments the more I felt that they proved the genuineness of the phenomena.

It is strange that with all this careful watching, no one ever discovered the trace of a trick in such clear and simple experiments, and many of us were most suspicious. And yet some sceptics say that if they had been there they would certainly have shown up the fraud, although all the witnesses were deceived! A well-known doctor was speaking about the phenomena of materialization observed by Dr. von Schrenk-Notzing, and said to me : " This does not exist for me, because I am a monist." I refuse to discuss the subject with such opponents and leave them to their " monism " ! We must accept the facts even if they are astounding and even if, at the start, we have no means of explaining them.

I will give my results in tabular form before going on to a general theoretical discussion of the subject. I take the experiments in which the results cannot possibly be put down to chance, even if the problem were not completely solved, as positive. It would not be fair to consider only the experiments in which everything was seen as positive, as we often broke them off, not intending everything to be read. We must also allow small mistakes (e.g. Zarastro instead of Sarastro), as even then the result is far beyond what could be put down to chance. This criterion is somewhat subjective in character, and yet it gives us the most correct picture. We have given feeble positive results " $\frac{1}{2}$ ".

TELEPATHY

No.	Object	Result		Observation
1	Shaving brush	Stopped	–	See p. 28
2	Scissors	Scissors	+1	See pp. 28, 29
3	Violin	Violin	+1	
4	Bottle	Bottle	+1	
5	Drawing : two squares and a triangle	Drawing : two squares and a triangle	+1	See Figs. 1, 2, p. 32

CLAIRVOYANCE

No.	Object	Result		Observation
6	Post card	Several words and picture recognized	+1	See Figs. 3, 4, 5, pp. 42, 43, 44
7	Post card	Several words and part of picture recognized	+1	See Figs. 6, 6a, 7, 7a, pp. 46, 47

EXPERIMENTS

No.	Object	Result		Observation
8	Box with cotton wool	Correct description of contents	+1	
9	" It is Thursday to-day "	" Wednesday past "	?	See pp. 49, 50
10	" Ja nje poni maju "	Meaningless syllables	+½	
11	" Jo anche pittore "	. . .	—	
12	26	26	+1	
13	100	100	+1	
14	" Athens is the capital of Greece "	" Athens "	+1	
15	" Sebald "	" Sebald "	+1	
16	"Absollon "	" Abholen "	+1	
17	434	434	+1	
18	231	231	+1	
19	987	—7	+½	[p. 57
20	" Eberhard "	" Eberhard "	+1	See Figs. 8, 9,
21	521	521	+1	Written
22	" München "	" München "	+1	See Figs. 10, 11
23	777	666 or 999	?	See p. 57
24	666 or 999	666 or 999	+1	See p. 57
25	" Faust "	" Faust "	+1	
26	" Wer nie sein Brot mit Tränen as "	" Brot "	+1	
27	" Barbara "	" Barbara "	+1	
28	21244	21244	+1	
29	" Agathe "	" Agathe "	+1	
30	" Happy is the man who can shut himself up from the world without hatred "	. . .	—	
31	" Freising "	" Freising "	+1	
32	" Mandoline "	" Mandoline "	+1	Writing did not tally
33	The drawing of a mouse	Approximately correct	+1	Figs. 12, 13, p. 61
34	" Helsingfors "	. . .	—	
35	" Madelene "	" Madelene "	+1	
36	" Arturo "	. . .	—	
37	" Carmen "	" Carmen "	+1	Writing good
38	" Panta rei "	" Panta rei "	+1	
39	" Ludwig Wilser " and some Sanskrit words	" Ludwig Wilser " and signs much like original	+1	Figs. 14, 15, p. 63
40	" Frommert "	" Anna or Unna "	—	
41	" Zacharias "	" Zacharias "·	+1	
42	" Sarastro "	" Zarastro "	+1	
43	" Cannstadt "	" Cannstadt "	+1	Figs. 16, 17, p. 63
44	" Pater "	" Pater "	+1	
45	824	Six or seven letters	—	

No.	Object	Result	Observation	
46	. . .	negative	–	
47	. . .	negative	–	
48	. . .	negative	–	
49	. . .	negative	–	
50	" Julius "	" Julius "	+1	
51 to 63	. .	negative	12–	
64	54	" As if connected with medicine "	?	See p. 66
65	844	. . .	–	
66	. . .	negative	–	
67	. . .	negative	–	
68	318	a " 1 " with a dot	–	
69	" To love is to suffer "	. . . . . .	–	automatic writing
70	18437	. . .	–	automatic writing
71	. . .	negative	2–	
72	. . .	negative	2–	
73	" Bern "	Parts of the image formed reproduced correctly	+½	See p. 67
74	934	907, 987, there is a 9	+½	
75	379	negative	–	
76	" Carmen "	negative	–	
77	821	8—1—3, etc.	+½	See p. 69
78	" Planegg "	a number, 1 and 6 or 0 ?	–	
	see 176th experiment		p. 139	

I must refer the reader to the experimental records and to the commentaries if he wants to form a judgment on the details, as these can hardly be given in tabular form, e.g. the copying of writing, etc. (Nos. 79–183.)

The same holds good to a greater degree for the experiments on psychoscopy, so it is no use tabulating them, and I must refer the reader to the text (p. 70).

I may further summarize a few more numerical relations. We have 183 experiments before us, 5 of which deal with telepathy. Among the 74 recorded experiments on cryptoscopy we have 1 with Miss Sch., 3 with Miss von B., 69 with Re, and 1 with H. (No. 176.) If in considering the experiments with Re I leave out those of the second period (Nos. 45–78), as Re was quite out of practice, and his clairvoyant faculty was disappearing rapidly (he only had a flash of it in

No. 50), we find 35 experiments. If we neglect the
two curious experiments (Nos. 23 and 24) we find 26
positive, 2 partly positive ($\frac{1}{2}$), 4 without any result,
and 1 wrong (No. 40). Nos. 23 and 24 are difficult to
gauge, we might consider No. 23 + 1 and No. 23 + $\frac{1}{2}$;
as the latter was only within the range of probability
for two slips ; but I prefer to leave them out altogether.
(It would have given us 27+, 3 + $\frac{1}{2}$, 1 −, and 4 unsolved.)
Truly a good result. We could add 1+, and 3 + $\frac{1}{2}$ out
of the second period.

With regard to the psychoscopic experiments, there
were 104 of them (Nos. 79 to 175, and 177 to 183).
If I neglect the experiments with Mrs. W., and Mr. Sch.,
which were only mentioned in an appendix, we have
100 experiments, 47 of which can be taken as positive,
if we want to be very critical we shall have to reduce
this number by 8 or 10, but that still gives us 30–40
per cent positive. Unfortunately I failed to note
whether or not the objects were known in the negative
experiments, or only did so from No. 105 on ; this
leaves us 73 experiments, of which 39 were " unknown "
and 34 " known ". We can take 9 to 12 of the former
as positive, and 18 to 23 of the latter, so it would seem
that the " known " were more successful, which would
speak in favour of telepathy ; but I think we must
not be too quick in concluding this, as chance may
influence the result very strongly in so small a number
of experiments ; if we take another part of this series
(that carried out in presence of Professor Gruber) we
get quite a different result.

This is the longest series of experiments carried out
with any member of the medical commission, and I
never knew the contents of the parcels, so that I could
not give any conscious or unconscious help to H.
I would remind the reader that neither Gruber nor any
other member of the commission gave any help to H.
during the experiments. If we take this series of
experiments, conducted under specially stringent and

exact conditions, we find that out of the 26 experiments we have 61·5 per cent positive if we judge them leniently or 46·1 per cent if we judge them very severely.

Thirteen of them were " unknown ", of which 8 to 6 were positive ; whereas 13 were " known ", of which 8 to 5 were positive. Here there is no indication that the " unknown " were more successful than the " known ", so that they speak against telepathy taking an important part. It is certainly not due to chance that 46 to 61 per cent of the experiments were positive, and we could expect a higher percentage still if all the disturbing factors have been eliminated.

III

ON THE THEORY OF TELEPATHY AND CLAIRVOYANCE

A. Criticism of the Physical Theory

I AGREE with Hopp when he says that the time to proceed to form theories for these phenomena has not yet come, although I profoundly disagree with his opinion of the material we already have at our disposal. Hence, if I go into the theory of the matter here, it is because other investigators have done so in such a way that the method used and the consequences they derive from it seem to me equally open to criticism. It would also appear that a preliminary theoretical discussion might give us valuable indications for the future, both as to how to judge experiments and how to plan them. Chowrin's work seems a case in point. Chowrin assumed at the very beginning of his work that these faculties depended on hyperæsthesia of the senses, and appears not to have seen any other possibilities. So that his experiments, which were in many ways very good, are all planned in one particular direction, and their results might have been turned to much better account if considered with an open mind. Schrenck-Notzing, who translated and edited his book, mentions this fact at the end of the book (see my comments in *Psychische Studien*, 1919, Nos. 10 and 11, pp. 547–50). When criticizing a piece of work it is natural for one to give positive indications of other ways in which the phenomena might be explained.

Science has a justifiable tendency to connect all the different sciences with one another, and to fill the gaps with hypothetical explanations. But this tendency should not lead scientists to make light of, or to ignore, any difficulties which might argue against these hypotheses ; on the contrary, these previsions should only be made after all the facts have been duly considered and taken into account. Often, this was not done, and facts which bore superficial analogies to one another were linked up into an hypothesis before a careful analysis of the facts had proved that they were really connected. Wireless telegraphy and the X-rays suggest themselves very strongly as analogies to telepathy and clairvoyance ; and they have often been used as an explanation of them ; but *the proof that we are in the presence of more than simple analogies has never been furnished with the necessary clearness and thoroughness.*

The scientist, naturally, tries to apply to the new study the conceptions which have helped him hitherto, but it is questionable whether they will cover the field, and this cannot be judged a priori, or assumed, but has to be tested by exact analysis of the facts. It is not at all certain whether natural science is right when it claims to be the only universal scientific language. Certainly, its field is a wide one, but if it crosses its borders and continues to ask questions in its own language, in all simplicity, it may receive answers which remind us of Hebbel's " Kannitverstan ", a well-known peasant who asked the dwellers of a foreign land questions in his own tongue, and thought that the " Kannitverstan " (" Can't understand ") he received in reply, was an intelligent answer, and so got a picture of things which varied considerably from the truth. The questions put, and the experimental order, have to be made to fit the nature of the field of investigation, and not all the results can be interpreted in one's own language ; for, just as it is unsuitable to investigate optical problems with apparatus used for sound, so we might find it unsuitable to try to read the book of psychics in physical language. At any rate it will be wise to see if there is not another script in another

tongue which shines through as in the ancient palimp-
sestes and may give us much more valuable information
than the writing on the surface.

Psychics is one of the fields in which the natural
scientist likes to apply his theories with a naïve conse-
quentiality ; he assumes without any epistemological
or psychological qualms that the psychical—which
does not exist in space—will follow the mechanical
laws of space, and builds airy hypothetical structures
for that purpose (see e.g. Verworn : *Die Mechanik
des Geisteslebens*, Leipzig, 1919, 4th ed. E. Becher
treats the subject much more profoundly in his book :
Gehirn und Seele, Leipzig, 1911).

The natural scientist is just as fond of waving his
sceptre over occultism and the phenomena of telepathy
and clairvoyance as of waving it over psychics.[1]

The attempt to try to find some " psychic force " to
explain these phenomena is not new (we may recall
Crookes and Schindler), and nearly every kind of wave
or vibration has been invoked for that purpose ;
magnetic waves, electric, electro-magnetic, odic rays,
ultra-red, ultra-violet, Röntgen rays, Radium emanations, N-rays, and several others have all had their
turn in explaining either telepathy or clairvoyance.
The most popular are wireless telegraphy as an explanation of telepathy, and X-rays as an explanation of
clairvoyance. Such an abundance of different explanations should encourage research and cause inquiry into
the conditions these different rays would require, in
order to produce the reactions demanded of them.
But this has only been done very summarily, and this
information is generally given in a purely general
statement.

I shall treat telepathy and clairvoyance separately,
not because I think that they are fundamentally
different, but without any preconceived opinion or

[1] In *Monismus and Okhultismus*, Leipzig, 1921, I go into the
epistemological and general theoretical fundamentals.

theory, simply because they have the external difference that in telepathy the action is of mind on mind, whereas in clairvoyance the action is between mind and an object (matter).

We may begin with the theory of *Telepathy*. This has always been compared with our other means of understanding—less so with language than with the technical devices of transmitting news at a distance (telephone and wireless telegraphy). These we must proceed to analyse.

Let us first consider speech. As Staudenmaier said quite rightly, we transmit news to one another through speech, which is " wireless ", so that it is really quite superfluous to look so far for a comparison. But why is speech not more used for this purpose ? First of all because it is too well known, however wonderful it may be ; but there may be another cause as well. Everybody is perfectly familiar with speech, and knows that conventional signs are the very basis of it. When we think of wireless telegraphy we are apt to forget that, or not to lay such weight on it, since the fact which strikes us most about it is that there is no material connexion as in speech or in ordinary telegraphy. But this absence of conventional signs is an essential point of difference between wireless telegraphy and telepathy.

Let us go a little deeper in our analysis of speech, and see how the " thought-transference " takes place. Let us suppose that I have an idea, and that I want to transmit it to someone else ; this idea is connected with certain processes in my brain, or, if I wish to transmit it, with processes in the speech-centres from which certain impulses pass to my speech-organs (mouth, larynx, etc.). Here, certain combinations of sounds will be emitted which will reach the ears of the person with whom I wish to communicate, as sound waves ; these waves will excite the auditory nerves, and the impulses thus formed will reach the hearer's brain, and there give rise to certain processes which will cause him to have the perception of sounds, etc. To these sounds there corresponds a certain " meaning " ; the " words " used by the speaker are " understood " and a " thought-transference " has taken place.

The comparison is very good, and it is surprising that it should not have been taken as a comparison instead of wireless telegraphy, especially as we are much better acquainted with speech. No doubt it was realized that telepathy was something quite different, and that we gain nothing by this comparison.

But we must analyse this means of communication by speech still more closely. How are these sound-waves, etc., transformed from thought into nerve-impulses ? Is it an automatic mechanical process, one which takes place with the same inevitability as any chemical or physical change, for instance a process which entails a caloric change, chemical change, the production of light, sound, and movement, say, by a machine or an explosion ? No, it is a different kind of process. The relation between the idea and the formation of sound waves in which the words which are to carry the idea are formed, is a matter of convention. The relation between the thoughts and the sound waves or sounds and their correspondence depends on artificial codes which are different in every language. In these languages the single ideas correspond with definitely chosen combinations of sounds, words, or we can say that a definite word has been allotted to each idea. These words are composed of combinations of sounds which are made up of comparatively few elements—for the sake of simplicity we will call them letters straight away—which have the power of expressing a great number of ideas owing to the great number of different combinations which can be formed out of them. We thus find that words are allotted to ideas and that these differ in the different languages, so that they have to be learned afresh in every language.

Later on, writing was originated for the transmission of these words to a distance and for their preservation. The combinations of sounds which form the words were analysed into their constituents—I am only considering the modern languages—which always kept recurring, and these elements were given certain signs, combinations of lines, which were to represent them permanently. So we have another completely different translation or remoulding from the spoken language to the written language, which is based on the differences in the acoustical and optical peculiarities, and has to form a suitable transition from one to the other. The sound " e " has nothing to do with the letter " e " intrinsically, it is a pure matter of convention. The written language requires the eye to take it in ; there are other possibilities of transmission. For instance, the heliograph, but this requires an apparatus which is sensitive to light, too. The Morse code and the Braille type are similar to these, in principle.

We may certainly assume that the person who deciphers the message in telepathy is, on the whole, passive, and that the other is active, although this has not yet been proved ; let us call them percipient and agent respectively. On the physical theory then, we should have an emission of rays or vibrations going from the brain of the agent, passing through his skull and his skin, through the intervening space, then through the skin and skull of the percipient to produce impulses, and images in his brain. So here, too, we should expect a system of signs, for it is not clear how such a transmission, which involves conversion of ideas into vibrations and conversion of vibrations into ideas, can take place without some system of signs. Waves travelling through space are not ideas according to physical theory ; at most they might be correlated with them, so that it would at the very least require a conversion by the agent and one by the percipient. We have no trace of these conversions, for we are not considering conjuring tricks here, but true telepathy. The phenomenon appears as the gradual apparition of an image out of a deep blue or nebulous background, auditions, intuition, or simply a feeling of a certainty of knowledge of the words. But, apart from this, there is no organ of transmission or of perception known, such as we have in speaking or in reading, and there is no part of the brain which could be thought to be one. But it seems hardly possible that such complicated results should be obtainable without some special organ ; yet it would be strange to find that a special organ should have been formed for so rare a faculty. Then again, there are no indications that it is a voluntary transformation and transmission such as we find in writing and speech.

It is certainly not a simple matter, and it will require some thought to get to the bottom of it. It may be said that it is not a voluntary conversion, but might be an automatic one like the conversions of sound into electro-magnetic waves and vice versa in the telephone, so that these two changes in the brain would be quite automatic ; but there is one difference, the conventional signs are sent into the telephone before the automatic change takes place, and to prove the possibility of this theory being correct we should therefore have to show that the telephone could transmit ideas without using a code of any sort. It is most probable that there are certain movements of the molecules, atoms, or electrons in the cells of our brains which correspond to these ideas—we do not know anything definite on the subject—and these movements or vibrations will vary with the different mental processes, but we cannot assume that they are so clearly defined and rhythmical as to be combined into a unit which entirely represents the process in the cell and thus to be considered as carrying the message of themselves. The rays emitted by a light or a fire are not so complex and so differentiated that they can transmit thought as such; it is only after they have been moulded and differentiated and arranged in a conventional code that they can be used for such a purpose.

Let us take a concrete example to see what this theory really would require. Let us suppose that a simple drawing of a cross in a circle is to be transmitted by telepathy. The agent will try to form a definite and clear image of the picture in his head. There will be a corresponding activity in the ganglia of his brain. How are we to picture these to ourselves? Modern brain-physiologists say that for every simple conception, at least eight ganglion cells come into action. So we can take, as a minimum, one ganglion cell for the cross and one for the circle. How shall we have to picture the transmission of the cross in this case? Is there a special kind of vibration for a cross or does the vibration itself have the shape of a cross? It may be said that the question itself sounds ridiculous, but we must ask it. Again, it is very doubtful whether the conception of a cross only requires the excitation of one single ganglion cell. But if the details of the cross are transmitted by different cells, where does the synthesis of these vibrations into a "cross in a circle" take place? We can only look for the factors of this synthesis in the vibrations; the brain of the recipient cannot help to combine them, as it can know nothing whatever of the object; but how is this synthetic function transmitted?

It seems obvious that the solution of the dilemma cannot be found in this direction. The eye does not come into the question as an image-forming organ; so that we should have to look for a similar organ in the brain—for this seems the only possible way of transmitting the synthetic unity of the picture. We should have to look for an organ constructed after the manner of an eye, a pin-hole camera, the compound eye of an

insect or Korn's telescope ; but no such organ has yet
been found. It is no use to say that some such organ
of a known or unknown design will perhaps be found ;
whoever frames such wild hypotheses must give sound
evidence for them. We may therefore say that neither
vibrations in the shape of a cross, nor the synthesis out
of elements, nor transmission by some yet undiscovered
organ, has been proved or is even conceivable.

This is but a preliminary question ! Now comes the
problem : how is this conceptual image to be transmitted to one definite cell of the visual centre ? As we
are speaking of vibrations or waves, the first answer
which suggests itself is that the two brains might be
tuned, so that one cell in the one should vibrate when
the corresponding cell in the other brain vibrates, like
the strings of two instruments which are tuned to the
same note. Now a ganglion cell is not a cord, and it is
difficult to conceive that there should be only one kind
of vibration in any one ganglion cell, which could be
projected from it like the sound from a string. But
even if this were the case, we cannot avoid the question ;
how are these waves converted into the corresponding
vibrations of the corresponding ganglion cells without
the presence of some complex organ of reception ? It
is possible to conceive that the correspondence between
ideas and brain-processes is strictly defined, parallel,
automatic, and completely reversible in different
individuals, although this may present some intellectual difficulties. But we should have to presuppose
that every single ganglion cell in the brain had its own
particular vibrations and that these particular vibrations should be the same for the corresponding cell "
every other brain. If this were not the case there would
be a fearful confusion : suppose, for instance, that
some other cell should vibrate at the same time in
one or the other of the two brains in communication.
I think that we can regard this as most improbable,
and conclude that a theory with so many and such

strong objections can be neglected till we have potent evidence in its favour.

So we must continue our search. What if we supposed that the two brains were absolutely similarly constituted, so that any point in the one should correspond to a point in the other, as do a point of a slide and a point of the projected image in magic-lantern pictures. In this way the image of the cross could be transmitted. But such a correspondence would not agree with the facts.

When I look at a cross to transmit it, a small image of the cross is formed on the retina of my eye. But this is not transferred to my brain ; this image is only the material my brain uses to form the idea of that cross. We do not find an image of that cross anywhere in the brain, and even if the cells excited in the retina were to excite a number of cells similarly arranged in the brain, we should have a cross of stimulated cells, not the image of a cross which would be transmitted to the second brain. So this very crude conception also fails to give us a clue.

We must remember that we have made a number of suppositions which are much too strongly in favour of the physical theory. It is generally recognized that, even for simple concepts, more than one ganglion cell takes part in the process. This does not simplify matters for the physical theory.

It is pretty clear that the ordinary kinds of physical energy do not yield a satisfactory result. If with Ostwald we suppose the existence of psychic energy, the question has quite another aspect. It would carry us too far afield to go into this theory in detail, but a number of strong objections have been raised by philosophers against this new form of energy. We will only just glance at things from this point of view and see where it leads us in occultism. In energetics everything is reduced to energy ; the only thing which exists is energy. Ostwald reduces matter to energy, and all psychic phenomena also. He thinks that the latter are due to the transformation of other forms of energy into nervous energy, and " psychic energy ". So it follows that psychic phenomena are not connected with or dependent on, or parallel to, any " energic " phenomena ; the idea itself is simply a form of energy, an " energetic " process, a certain amount of " pyschic energy ", and nothing more, for nothing exists except energy.

If we apply these theories to the problems in hand, we find the following possibilities ; psychic energy must either be bound to the ganglion cells or be free. In the first case we have much the same proposition as above ; we should have to explain how it is transformed, transmitted, received, and reconverted into conceptions.

We have seen how great are the difficulties in this case, and we need not repeat them. In the second case, where no transformation is needed and the energy simply goes from the agent to the recipient through space, we have the following points to consider. The ideas are energy according to this hypothesis, so we must conclude that they are transmitted as such, not that they are bound up with some psychic vibration which represents them or which is closely connected with them ; they would then be *vibrations* or *rays* which would pervade space as such. That is, we should have to conclude that a psychic " something " existed quite apart from our bodies, a something which would have a free existence of its own in space. I think that the naturalists and positivists would be the first to find this odd and refuse to accept it. It is hard to explain how this idea travels, how and where it takes hold of the individual so as to enter his consciousness, or is a part of " consciousness ". Does the synthesis first formed travel unaltered as a whole through space, or how is it built up from its elements ? All these questions are more easily asked than answered.

TELEPATHY AND CLAIRVOYANCE

The problem of clairvoyance is of rather a different nature, as the " agent " is not a second person but a thing. Here, too, the natural scientist is more likely to suppose that rays of some sort pass from the object to the clairvoyant, and act upon him in some way. So we must suppose that rays emanated from the post card, " ink-rays," which permeate the black paper and the other coverings. By analogy we shall have to conclude that there are rays of cotton wool which can permeate paper and cardboard. In one of Wasielewski's experiments we find a small metal case with cotton wool and a " small hollow thing made of yellow metal, not gold " ; this was recognized. We must therefore suppose that all these things emit special rays : that the " cotton wool rays " go through metal and the " metal rays " through cotton wool and other metals ; that these different rays do not interfere with one another in the least, and that not only the colour and substance of the particular object but even its form were more or less recognized. Ink, graphite, paper, and many other rays have been recognized, whereas such rays have never been detected in physics. It might be supposed that this recognition was not supersensual, but took place through the eye. There are many objections to this supposition. First of all the existence of the rays has not been proved. Then there are certain observations which Wasielewski published in his book on Telepathy and Clairvoyance which do not seem to be explicable in this way, especially some of the cases of clairvoyance at a distance. Some of the things recognized were so small that they were below the range of sight. Helmholtz has shown that the mosaic of the retina only gives us the possibility of distinguishing two points when they are at least one minute apart, angular measure. To distinguish smaller objects than that is no more possible to the unaided eye than it is to put gravel through a duster. So we cannot claim that clairvoyance takes place through the eye or through any other sense organ ; but then we encounter the same difficulties as in telepathy ; we know of no organ through which it can take place. The problem of how the vibrations reaching the brain are taken up and transformed is not yet solved.

If we consider the experiments with Miss von B. in connexion with the theory of rays of psychic energy, experiments in which words were read and even written with many of the chief characteristics of the original writing, we are again led to ask how it is possible to receive such waves and convert them without a suitable organ for that purpose, especially as there is no possibility of a corresponding arrangement of cells as in telepathy, and there obviously can be no parallelism between the structure of the brain and that of the object.

Wasielewski once gave Miss von B. an envelope containing a sheet of paper, with writing only on one side, which she held against her forehead ; she read it correctly holding it with the writing on the side of the paper next her head. She turned the paper. When the writing was on the far side, one would have expected her to see the writing converted in a looking-glass, but she saw it just as she had seen it before. This one experiment already speaks very strongly against the physical theory, as the rays emanating from the letter should then have caused a different result in both cases.

The reading of folded slips by Re is still more interesting from that point of view. It we try to explain them by the physical theory, we must remember that, as we said before, the letters overlap and the slip would only give a medley of lines if it were seen as through the paper. This experiment proves definitely that the sight cannot take place through the eyes, and is a fact *which weighs very heavily against any physical explanation* ; for it is quite inconceivable that the rays coming from the slip could possibly be analysed in such a way that the slip could be seen spread out flat, if these rays were perceived parasensorially. This chaos of lines cannot be deciphered, and even if we suppose that it could be deciphered after much practice, it is not clear why this should not be possible when the slip is being looked at in the normal way, yet Meyer proved that this is never the case.

Another way in which the process might be supposed to take place—rather a vague one—is that rays should be emitted by the clairvoyant—" brain waves "—to the object, and should be reflected by the object back to him and give him information about it. This process would be similar to that used by the blind, who gain a knowledge of their surroundings by the reflection of sounds ; as we sometimes do in the dark to find out the size of a room and the presence of obstacles. Some persons have developed this faculty to a degree which allows them to gauge very accurately the size and distance of objects in their vicinity. But these are very vague and fantastic surmises to base clairvoyance on. It is not clear how these reflected rays could give information not only about the size and shape of the object, but also about the material it is made of. In this case, also, we do not know the organ of perception.

We adduced the fact of clairvoyance at a distance in opposition to the theory that the action took place through the eye, but it is a very potent argument against any form of rays causing the phenomena. How can we suppose an object to project rays which enable a clairvoyant to recognize it hundreds of miles away ; how can we explain the fact that one of thousands of persons at such a distance should be seen doing some particular thing at the moment he is doing it ? Even reflected brain waves do not help to explain it. The projecting apparatus would have to be very powerful indeed to project the waves to such a distance ; and how would they come back, or what organ would perceive them ?

THEORY

We have seen that the ray theories do not explain either telepathy or clairvoyance. The only theory which might yet fit the case is the corpuscular theory. We should have to imagine that minute particles are emitted by the objects, say electrons, and that these carry the necessary information, but this seems improbable. Either the electrons are in vibration, and the problem is the same as before, or we suppose that the electrons themselves are the bearers, and we find ourselves facing one of the greatest problems of philosophy, i.e. how is matter converted into ideas? a problem which the materialist solves with ease by saying that the idea accompanies matter or is a function of it, unless he goes so far as to say that it is a product of it, statements which are not in accord with the nature of the psychical.

So-called transference of the senses, in which the medium reads with the tips of the fingers, or with the pit of the stomach, the feet, etc., is a problem which can hardly be solved by any physical theory.[1] The physical theory would require the presence of a suitable organ of sense at the place where the sensation is located, and this seems most improbable. Now if, as is sometimes the case, these zones are centres of hearing, smell, etc., as well as sight, we shall have to assume that a universal organ exists at that point, a fact which, I fancy, can hardly be brought into accordance with our physical and physiological knowledge.

Now; a few words about the psychoscopic experiments. There have been several attempts to explain them by physical hypotheses or conceptions. Kotik spoke of " psychic energy ", Böhm of a " psychic coating" which should stick to the object, and both were thinking in pure physical terms. But here, too, physical theories are not of much use, as we cannot

---

[1] An interesting attempt to construct such a theory on a histological basis has, however, recently been made by M. Jules Romains (Louis Farigoule) in his *Eyeless Sight*, London, 1924. [*Trans.*]

find out how these physical traces can possibly cause such complex incidents, feelings, etc., to be perceived. The theoretical considerations are just the same as in pure clairvoyance, so I need not go over them again in detail. This point of view does not cover the ground if we really think in terms of physics and do not tie psychic properties to our energies, contrary to all physical tradition.

I have discussed the ray theory very thoroughly, and we need not go into it in further detail. I would only mention the attempts to find organs which might be sensitive to these rays. Among those most frequently supposed to have this property is the solar plexus, an agglomeration in the neighbourhood of the pit of the stomach. Mediums often hold the objects against the pit of their stomach, but I am inclined to think that this is simply an acquired habit which is not really connected with the perception in any way. It is no use to put the perception down to the action of the solar plexus in our case, as I do not see why it should act better, as a receptive and converting organ, than the brain. The same holds good for other organs which might be, or have been, regarded in the same way. Among these we find the pineal gland and the ganglions of the adrenal gland.

We will conclude with a few words on the distinction between telepathy and clairvoyance. The distinction made earlier in this work rests on the fact that the transmission takes place between two individuals in the former case, and between an object and an individual in the latter. The question is whether this distinction really touches a vital difference or is only an external characteristic. As we saw in telepathy we call one person the agent, the other the percipient ; and that is to say we suppose that the former takes an active part in the proceedings. Are we to suppose that this is the case when the percipient tells us about things of which the agent has not thought for a long time, things which he has forgotten all about, and that he can hardly call to mind even with a great effort, or even fails to remember at all ? If we make this activity of the agent the criterion of telepathy we must exclude the above-mentioned cases from it and refer them to the old idea of " soul-reading " (Schindler, Perty) or to " mind-reading " in the true sense of the word. It is hard to tell whether we should consider this mind-reading as belonging to clairvoyance or to telepathy. It has this in common with telepathy : that they are both connected with knowledge of the content of the mind. It is comparable to clairvoyance, for in both cases the same agent seems to be active and the other person or thing, passive, so that the so-called " agent " is as passive as a thing. So thought-reading has important characteristics in common with both and it may be that purely practical considerations should guide us in making the distinction. The faculty of some mediums (Aub for instance) would have to be classed as mind-reading. Psychologists who deny the existence of the subconscious mind will recognize these two classes a priori, and take them as two distinct phenomena. But all those who do not regard the soul as the same thing as the mind will find it very practical to keep the two processes apart, regardless of certain intermediate cases which occur pretty frequently, in which the " agent " is more or less active. If we lay much weight on the fact that there is no definite line of distinction between " soul-reading " and telepathy we can class the former as a special type of the latter ; if we think that it is not the content of the mind but the brain-states and processes which are perceived and which give us the means of deciphering its contents as we decipher writing, then we shall have to classify it as coming under the heading of clairvoyance—for it would have the two chief characteristics of clairvoyance, the activity of one person only and clairvoyant perception of material processes. All these classifications

are somewhat schematic, for it is quite possible that
telepathy and clairvoyance are not two different things,
but two modifications of one of the basic faculties of
the mind ; this suggestion is supported by the fact that
they often appear mixed up in all sorts of ways. The
romantic school and I. H. Fichte spoke of a " universal
sense ". Wasielewski is of the same opinion ; he thinks
that they are different activities of a faculty which
he calls " panaesthesia ".[1]

B. Theoretical views of other Authors

I should like to mention the views of certain
modern authors. Ostwald is inclined to accept the
phenomena as genuine, but seems to have considered
the subject only in a general way. He says in a review
of one of Flammarion's books (*Annal. für Naturphil.*,
1910, vol. ix, p. 212) : " If we assume that persons
(or certain persons known as mediums) have the faculty
of transforming part of the energy which they have
in the form of chemical energy in their bodies and
which they generally turn into mechanical energy
through their muscles in such a way that it leaves their
bodies and can come into action at arbitrarily chosen
places ; if we concede this we have the necessary
premises for an explanation of these phenomena."
In *Forderung des Tages* (1910, p. 418), he writes :
" Certain persons have the faculty of transforming
their store of physiological energy (which is almost
exclusively in the form of chemical energy) into other
forms which they can project through space and trans-
form into one of the known forms of energy at given
points in space." It would seem that Ostwald accepts
this branch of knowledge because he thinks he sees
a way of explaining it by his " energetics ".

[1] Cf. F. H. W. Myers' use of the word, which he introduced. He
describes the undifferentiated sensory capacity of the supposed
primal germ by that term. Wasielewski uses it with a slightly
different and more general sense. [*Trans.*]

THEORY

Naum Kotik builds up his theories on Ostwald's " energetics ". He thinks that there is a " psychoscopic energy " which consists of two parts : the " brain-rays " which have a very high coefficient of permeability and the psychic part of the energy which has a very low one. He also calls the latter the " Emanation of psychophysical energy " and claims that " it can cause the exact reproduction of the ideas it was connected with in the brain of the thinker, in any brain into which it penetrates ".

Staudenmaier, too (*Die Magie als Experimentelle Wissenschaft*, Leipzig, 1912), thinks that telepathy is due to an excitation of the brain-centres " which produces vibrations in the surrounding ether which are transmitted for miles ". He is of the opinion that, " if I send my thoughts to another person by means of air-waves it is not different in principle from telepathy where I send them by waves of the ether." He regards as " mystical " the view that something purely mental is imparted to the other person.

I. Boehm expressed himself similarly in his early writings, but he has now altered his opinion so that it is not necessary to criticize his earlier views. He now thinks that these phenomena cannot be explained by physical theories.

M. Benedict (cf. my essay in the *Zentralbatt für Okkultismus*, 1919), and his pupil Scheminski, want to explain these phenomena by emanations ; they speak of " radiant pressure " and " antennial brain ", etc.; they think that the emanation is the same as Reichenbach's Od.

A. Forel (*Journ. für Psychol. und Neurol.*, 1918) seems to me to have given the best explanation of telepathy and clairvoyance up to now. He thinks that the emission of electrons transmits the messages, but says that it would be ridiculous to suppose that the electrons themselves give rise to the sensations, perceptions, and even abstract conceptions of the medium. He says that we must not forget that in every brain, especially the adult brain, there are a number of engram-complexes, and he fancies that under certain special conditions the electrons are perceived or felt by the medium. Of course the condition that the complexes of electrons of the agent (brain or object) should react on the correspondingly engraphized parts of the brain of the medium is a *conditio sine qua non*, and also that the engram-complexes and the electron-complexes would thereby be caused to vibrate "homophonously and synchronously" which would produce special sensations. He suggests experiments which should test his views. He says that if no optical phenomena can be transmitted to subjects who were born blind or who are only clairaudient, it would be in favour of his theory.

The only opponents of a purely physical explanation I shall mention are Wasielewski and Hopp. Wasielewski mentions the physical theories several times in his book, and discards them on much the same grounds as were discussed above—comparison with ordinary speech, absence of receptive organs, etc.—but without going into such detail. He draws particular attention to the fact that words were seen the right way round on a wrapped up card, whether it was held against the head of the medium with the writing towards her or on the opposite side. The fact that a mirror image was not seen in either case speaks very strongly against the physical theory.

Hopp draws attention to the fact that the properties of physical rays do not explain the production of two analogous conceptions in two different brains. It is not clear how these specific rays produce psychical reactions. Hopp did not go into the non-radiant theories as they were all put forward without any serious arguments.

It will have been noticed that Forel was the only exponent of the physical theories who went into details. No one mentions that codes of signals are used in speech and in wireless telegraphy, both of which are used as comparisons ; this alters the face of things altogether. No one tackles the difficulties of how the correspondence of the two brains is constituted or how the conversion from and to the rays takes place. No one ever tries to explain how complex things such as drawings may be transferred without a synthesis taking place, a thing which would be quite inexplicable by such theories. The difficulty of explaining the reading of folded slips escapes them altogether, so of course they do not try to solve it. Ostwald's psychic energy does not do all that is expected of it, not do Kotik's emanations ; the latter goes into considerable detail, but passes over the above points, and his theories cannot explain them.

Let us consider Forel's theory more in detail, as he works it out much more thoroughly. Forel would like to find a common explanation for telepathy and clairvoyance. If we accept his theory we should find that the same engram-complex would be excited in telepathy say by the transmission of the idea of a stone, as in clairvoyance by a hidden stone, i.e. the conception of a stone which would already be there ; this presupposes that the electron-complex coming from the other brain and from the stone must be exactly alike or else they would not be " homophonous and synchronous " and so excite the engram-complex ; this theory takes for granted that the concept stone will always be the same. We may regard this as most improbable; it is not at all obvious how the concordance of vibrations in such different cases as the idea of a stone and the radiations of a stone could occur.

Forel's theory only covers the cases in which the necessary engram-complexes are already there. The cases where that is not so, where, for instance, intricate designs which the medium has never seen are to be recognized, would be quite inexplicable. The synthesis and the comprehension of the reading of folded slips is quite incomprehensible according to this theory. (See my reply to Forel's paper in the *Zeitschr. für Psychotherapie und Medizin. Psychologie*, 1920.) If we review all these arguments, we find that the theory of radiations does not give us the necessary data to explain either telepathy or clairvoyance satisfactorily, so that it cannot be considered as the true explanation. *The recognition of composite drawings and the reading of folded slips in which the writing overlaps seem to me to justify our definitely rejecting the physical theories as possible explanations.*

It is not a sound scientific argument in favour of the physical theories to say that if these difficulties do not agree with the properties of *known* rays, they may be explicable by rays still *unknown*; for we can say nothing about their properties as yet. Prediction is always rather a delicate thing, but these rays would have to possess properties which do not fit into physical nature at all. Let us see what are the conditions these rays would have to fulfil. Rays would have to be emitted by the overlapping writing, which would make it come out in perfect sequence in the mind of the medium, for we have seen that the brain is not capable of deciphering this general muddle of lines. But unless we endow these physical rays with purely psychological properties, we cannot expect them to possess a mental faculty like the one required to exhibit this mixture of lines arranged rationally as if the slip lay unfolded in front of the seer. I think we may be allowed to consider that as most improbable ; it is really too far fetched and much more fantastic and surprising than the facts themselves. The same thing applies to telepathy ; the brain cannot synthesize an abstract drawing ; it can get no clues as to the nature of the required synthesis from rays emitted by the object. Here, too, the absorbed rays would have to take intelligent control of the brain. So we are faced by the intellectual rays again. Physics would surely pronounce its own doom if it made such concessions.

Physics must face these facts and set to work seriously ; it must not be content with the hope that the future may make it all right. Physical theories can only expect to command attention when they have mastered all these difficulties and explained them satisfactorily in detail *by purely physical means*. They cannot expect to be treated seriously till that has been done. Telepathy is not explained by a simple allusion to wireless telegraphy.

The reader must not be misled into believing that I claim that no connexion exists between radiant energy and occultism. I fancy radiant energy will render great services in explaining phenomena in another field of occultism which does not concern us here. I would only protest against the absolute derivation of all psychic phenomena from the realm of physics only, and the vague and general manner in which the problems under consideration are treated by it. I do not deny the presence of little known or unknown rays which emanate from living beings, particularly from the human brain. It may be already proved that they are stronger when the person thinks (Kotik, Kilner) ; but these facts do not yet prove the presence of " thought rays ", they only prove that thought is accompanied by the physical processes—increased circulation in the brain and physical-chemical processes in the substance of the brain—which cause the production or increase of such rays.

C. A Psychical Theory

But is this all that knowledge can tell us ? Perhaps another method may lead us further ; at any rate it is our duty to try every path which might lead us to our goal. Is it really the obvious thing to try to explain telepathy and clairvoyance by physics at all costs ? [1]

We need not embark on a long epistemological inquiry,[2] but can say that the processes which are observed both in the agent and percipient are of what we call a " psychic " nature. We can, of course, try to reduce it to physical terms, but then we are putting an *interpretation* on it which is open to discussion. It is illogical to ignore the psychical from the start and only to speak of it in terms of physics ; such a thing as the psychical does exist.

The tendency is to try to class the psychical in the realm of matter. Materialism says it is due to movements of matter without trying to prove this in any way. But this is a purely verbal solution, and would take us too long to refute.

Ostwald's " energetics " have replaced materialism in the minds of many scientists. I have already spoken of them at some length in connexion with particular aspects of the question. But I must supplement my previous statements with a few more general considerations. The other forms of energy are mutually convertible in absolutely definite quantitative relations called " equivalents ". A definite quantity of heat-energy is equivalent to a definite amount of chemical energy. We know nothing comparable with this in psychics ; psychical energy has never been measured, so that we cannot possibly speak of a quantity of psychical energy, and no equivalents with other energies are known. But there are other ways in which the psychical

---

[1] Before entering the realm of metaphysics, we must emphasize that all our previous considerations have been purely empirical, and have had as little or as much to do with metaphysics as when a physicist decides, as a result of his experiments, against or in favour of the atomic theory of heat, or the wave theory of light. So that even if what now follows should later prove to be untenable, it will not reduce the value of the previous considerations in the least.

[2] For greater detail, see my *Monismus und Okkultismus*, Leipzig, 1911.

does not fit in with our conception of energy. Energies are bound to space, we measure the amplitudes of their vibrations, etc.; and all questions of space are ridiculous here, for we cannot go into the length and breadth of an idea. We can reduce energies to a few factors ; in psychics the further we go the greater is the number of facts we find which cannot be referred to one another. We have the actual content, and also knowledge about that content ; this relation of the actual content and to the knowledge about it is a thing absolutely unknown in " energetics ", and we do not see how to express such a relation in terms of energies. In fact, the two are so fundamentally different in every way that we can say that to speak of " energy " is to use a habitual word for a totally different thing. If, then, the psychical cannot be referred to the physical, let us consider the psychical in itself in connexion with the problems under consideration ; and let us proceed by keeping to a comparison of the observed facts and the direct conclusions to be drawn from them rather than soaring into the sky of theory.

Bergson has come to the conclusion that our memories are not located in the brain. He came to this conclusion by a profound study of certain lesions of the brain, which led to aphasia (loss of the power of speech). He found that it was a kind of switchboard, and that the reminiscences were stored up in the " pure memory ", i.e. in the mind.

The philosopher, Erich Becher, has studied the same problem in his book *Gehirn und Seele*, in which he investigates it in a series of very cleverly planned experiments and a chain of well thought out arguments. He proves that a memory due to purely physical traces left in the ganglia of our brains is inexplicable, and shows that we must assume the presence of purely mental memory-traces which are not bound in any way to the brain and do not correspond to the changes in the ganglia ; these we must regard as independent factors which are not necessarily in correspondence with the brain. We must assume the same thing for other psychical processes as we have been led to accept for memory, the standard example of the psycho-physiologists, and often to a much greater extent.

So we seem to be justified in leaving the old ground of psycho-physiology for the explanation of the facts of our everyday life, and looking further afield for the necessary explanations.

Now that Becher has proved that the facts of memory are not explicable by the theories of a mechanistic psycho-physiology, that we are forced to go further and conclude that a physical process does not accompany every mental manifestation, and that all mental processes are not in direct and inseparable connexion with the processes and residues in the brain, we feel justified in accepting, nay we have to accept, the possibility or even probability of other purely mental or psychical processes which are not absolutely dependent on the brain. *We are thus led by a series of exact experiments to assume, at least in principle, the possibility of the action of the mind outside the body, e.g. from one person to another, and that directly, as in the transference of thought.*

So the foundations of a psychical theory of telepathy and clairvoyance have been laid. But before taking the leap and assuming the direct action of one mind on another we may consider the possibility of the action of the *brain* of the agent on the *mind* of the percipient, which seems an obvious and at the same time a smaller step. Many scientists think that the brain of an individual has an action on his mind, but it is clear that the assumption that the brain of the agent acts on the mind of the percipient does not help us any further. The difficulties we met with in considering the applicability of the physical theories are still there, especially the most important, the explanation of the synthesis of composite drawings in telepathy. This explanation could not apply to clairvoyance.[1]

The only possibility left is a " mind theory ", i.e. a theory which supposes that transmission in telepathy and the acquisition of information in clairvoyance are purely *mental phenomena*; and that these must, of course, be distinguished from the way in which this information *becomes conscious* in a normal healthy brain.

I will refrain from going into details. It is very difficult to say anything definite about these in the realm of the mind, since our language was made for communication about the spatial and sensual world. It must be mentioned that the objections and difficulties which we encountered in trying to find a physical explanation disappear completely, or nearly so, when we come to deal with them in this way. We need no organs of emission or perception. Let us picture to ourselves the working of the mind say in lifting an arm ; the mind needs no sense organs to know how or where to excite the muscles. This very crude example shows us how the mind may work outside the body ; it may give us a very rough but sufficient analogy. We might suppose that the mind would use much the same methods to recall a residue out of the mental memory, and to catch a message which another mind had sent through space, and to call up the same image as the

---

[1] The difficulty seems to be that the brain would have to project itself or to send out power which would act directly on the impulses and sense organs of the other person. In this case the phenomenon would be material, not mental or psychical. We have an example of a similar phenomenon in the control of arms and hands in automatic writing and the control of mediums in trance. But is it a brain which causes these phenomena or a mind ? If a brain could gain control of another body or part of it at a distance, surely it could impart its power of conception to it, if this is regarded as due to chemical and other actions in that brain. This would explain the transmission of composite drawings and other syntheses. But a living brain ceases to be able to control its own members when a nerve or a minute material connexion is destroyed ; how then should it control another body without a material connexion ? This and the facts of cryptoscopy and psychoscopy seem to be two of the greatest difficulties this theory would meet with. [*Trans.*]

agent had. The principle in clairvoyance is much the same, but it is very difficult to say anything about it in detail at present, though the way in which the information is revealed to the mind seems to be much the same in principle ; this holds good for cryptoscopy, spatial clairvoyance, and psychoscopy.

The mind, being a non-spatial entity, has quite a different relation to space ; this cannot only be conjectured, but stated as a fact on the strength of the reading of folded slips. Such ideas as we have of the spatial world on the strength of our physical constitution do not help us here, and we are forced to conclude that quite different spatial conditions exist between space and mind. It is possible that we shall be able to get more details about that experimentally. We shall never be able to have a clear conception of it, and we shall soon reach the limit of our mental life as conditioned by our brain. I would merely mention one other alternative, which seems still more fantastic. If we concede clairvoyance in time, it is possible that the reading of the folded slips would be due to the faculty of seeing them unfolded either before the experiment when they were being written or afterwards when they are being read.

Psychoscopic experiments have a particular attraction from a philosophical point of view ; for through them we seem to catch a glimpse of the workshop of the " World-mind "—to get a partial or disconnected view every now and then of the medley of disordered happenings of past and present with a limited and one-eyed vision. In other words, experiment seems to show that thoughts and words leave traces in the super-individual mind which can be recognized by the seer. These experiments remind us of Herbart's views, and still more of Czolbe's. He is of the opinion that perceptions have an individual existence on a sensual basis, like the atoms; we might suppose that they have an individual existence on an ideal or mental basis, in fact that they are mental atoms. Both these views are unsatisfactory, and so, as we saw, the attempt has been made to derive all clairvoyance from telepathy ; this cannot be regarded as a success. Psychoscopy is most problematic, and leads us on to quite fantastic lines if we start theorizing, so we had better turn back.

One thing more. These problems involve us in a consideration of Time. It certainly seems very strange when events long past and buried in the ashes of bygone years seem to creep up again. This appears not to be quite consistent with our conceptions of Time. We might try here to apply Kant's theory of the transcendental ideality of Time, i.e. its subjectivity. But apart from the fact that the transcendental realists will scarcely view it with a favourable eye, it is hard to see how it would make things clearer. It would simply be a confession that this question cannot be dealt with rationally, a conclusion at which we might arrive without the aid of Kant.

We might here mention the recent investigations of Einstein and Minkowski who regard Time as a fourth dimension. It is well known that space and time lose their absolute character in Einstein's theory of relativity ; everything becomes relative, as also the concepts " before ", " now ", and " after ", which are only true for a definite system. This seems to open the possibility of explanations and to hold out a hope that occultism may lose some of the strangeness that accompanies it. I cannot go into these questions here ; they would lead us into the domain of higher mathematics. It is even possible that the very occultism which is so looked down upon will one day be used as a proof for the theories of the most modern mathematicians and physicists. But this cannot be judged until the mathematics of this field of research have been thoroughly explored. If this fails there are other possibilities of trying to understand these phenomena.

TELEPATHY AND CLAIRVOYANCE

Both opponents and supporters of occultism are inclined to think that here we have reached the limit of reason ; that occultism is not rationally explicable. I do not agree with them. I fancy that there are large parts of it which we may be able to explain just as rationally as physics and physiology, but we may really have come to a point where some things are not explicable by our manner of thought, which is only suited to the world of space and time, and we shall thus be moving in the irrational. Only the dogmatist who knows a priori that the world is a rational creation can deny this. Others will consider this possibility and try to become better acquainted with it.

We must look at these things from another angle. Supernormal phenomena are often produced in a state in which the consciousness of everyday life, the waking consciousness, has completely disappeared, and other strata of the mind, which are not accessible to us under ordinary circumstances, have taken command. Miss von B. and Re belong to the class of mediums who produce phenomena without any apparent change in their state of consciousness. Sometimes the former loses the synthetic faculty of our normal consciousness ; this can also be considered as being the case when she copies writing. The field of her waking consciousness would certainly seem to be narrowed down in these cases. Both of them adopted automatic writing very quickly, Re while I was watching him. This, too, points to the fact that their subconscious mind stood in an abnormal relation to their waking consciousness at the time ; so that part of it could readily split off. It is typical of persons with the gift of mediumship that they can recall long-forgotten events from the depth of their mind to their surface consciousness in different ways, e.g. by crystal-gazing, automatic-writing, trance-utterance ; and this often led the uncritical to ascribe the results to telepathy, clair-voyance, or even to the spirits of the departed, since they showed no knowledge of these facts in their waking state.

Apart from this subconscious memory, we find the same people giving us information really gained supernormally, which, as far as we can tell, seems to be connected with their subconscious minds in some way. As these mediums bring forth knowledge which does not belong primarily to the life of their individual minds, and which they cannot have gained through their senses, the idea suggests itelf that these strata stand in a different relation to things than does our waking consciousness. It gives us the impression that the subconscious mind—to make use of a spatial image— is not so clearly separated from its surroundings, but represents a mental field which is connected with the " non-individual " or super-individual mind. If we descend from our surface consciousness we gradually reach subconscious mental regions which cease to belong to a single individual—as when we follow a watercourse into the interior of a mountain we reach regions where we lose sight of the single stream but where water pervades the ground all around us. These very deep layers of the subconscious mind would thus share in a non-individual or super-individual mind and so have a knowledge of things which are quite unattainable and incomprehensible to the individual mind. The difficulty of raising this knowledge to the surface consciousness would account for the scarcity of these phenomena.

In clairvoyance, the individual has a knowledge of things which he has not obtained through his senses, and which he comes by in a way which seems quite mysterious to our understanding. It is only our own inner life which is known to us in this fashion ; we have a knowledge of it without the use of our senses. This is the only actual case in which we find the acquisition of knowledge without the use of our senses, and it is the only imaginable one. If we are not content to give up all hope of getting to know what really happens in clairvoyance, we must proceed from the known to the unknown, and try to grasp it, aiding ourselves with the similar cases we do know. It is not a very long step to take to consider these cases as related instead of only similar. So we should conclude that exactly as we ourselves have direct knowledge of the facts and states of our minds and in our minds, the clairvoyant has just the same knowledge of non-individual or super-individual mental contents which contain a knowledge of outside facts, events, feelings, etc. Two different trends of thought have brought us to the conclusion that the individual can claim a share in a super-individual or collective mind.

In his *Wirklichkeitslehre*, Driesch draws our attention to the fact that we only know mind empirically as an individual mind ; this individual mind is spread over different individuals as on islands. No bridges seem to go from one to·the other ; a conclusion which is most extraordinary, in fact, incomprehensible, if we had to accept it as final. If there is really a super-individual or collective mind, as we have tried to prove above, then this extraordinary isolation of the individual mind ceases to be so strange. For if we accept this hypothesis the individual mind will lose its isolation and it becomes comprehensible why the mind is so homogenous regardless of its isolation, and the origin of the individual minds would cease to be problematical as they would all come from the common reservoir.

Had I not found myself in agreement with other investigators, I should not have dared to indulge in speculations of this kind, lest I should be called a mystic, and not read at all. Most of these other investigators were following different paths and came to the same conclusion. E. von Hartmann, when speaking about telepathy, in much the same way refers to the " telephonic connexion with the Absolute ", and he thinks of individuals as in direct mental connexion with the Absolute. Again, we meet E. Becher with his views on the " super-individual mind ". Becher found in the course of careful scientific investigations on the gall of plants that the obvious fitness of this gall could not be explained by the Darwinian or Lamarckian theories, since it was incomprehensible why the plant should form an excrescence which was not of any use to itself, but to quite another organism. (E. Becher, *Die Fremddienliche Zweckmässigkeit der Pflanzengallen und die Hypothese eines über individuellen Seelischen,* Leipzig, 1917.) This " altruisic fitness " points to a super-individual factor, and he surmises that these far-sighted modifications are brought about by a very weak individual consciousness combined with a super-individual mind which projects its branches into the individuals.

A well-known neurologist, Kohnstamm (*Journal f. Psychol. und Neurol.*, 1918, Beiheft.), has lately tried to prove that in the deepest hypnosis a stratum is reached which is beyond the individuality and the personality. His subjects maintain that in the deepest hypnosis they can dive down to strata of their sub-conscious mind which are impersonal. The utterances of this deepest layer are of general applicability and no longer have to do with the person in question and his characteristics ; it might just as well apply to any-one else, as this subconscious mind always thinks objectively ; Kohnstamm maintains that he has reached the universal, pure, super-individual, absolute subject.

These views of Becher and Kohnstamm may or may not be accepted ; at any rate they agree very well with the results of our experiments and with our theoretical considerations, and they certainly facilitate the comprehension of the observations we have recorded. We can say that these phenomena might readily be *deduced*, nay *predicted*, from the super-individual mind and the absolute subject. For if the super-individual mind projects more or less deeply into every individual, it is not only comprehensible but *to be expected* that a mental connexion should exist between two individuals, just as two pipes which are joined to the same reservoir have a connexion between both their surfaces, which never leaves the liquid.

As already mentioned, these views may serve to make the facts more comprehensible. *The facts themselves are quite independent from the acceptance of the theoretical considerations of Becher and Kohnstamm.* I personally do not regard their views as proved, but as well worth consideration. We can, however, use them to help to render our psychic theory more comprehensible ; a supporter of Becher's theory will not find it difficult to accept. This view of the psychic theory seems to me a better argument in favour of the super-individual mind than Becher's, in that it makes the rival theories more untenable ; so that even an opponent of Becher's theory might find it worth considering. It seems to me that supporters of the theory of the interaction of body and mind should not find it hard to accept telepathy ; the path from mind to mind would no longer present a difficulty (if there were a direct telepathic connexion from mind to mind) since the physical intermediates would drop out. The most difficult problem for the supporters of that theory was the action of the mind on the body and vice versa ; the action of mind on mind never was a problem to them.

IV

CONCLUSION

IN conclusion a few remarks may be offered on points which need not be fully discussed here. It may help us to judge things in their true light.

I will not venture further into metaphysics, and would only add that I do not pretend to explain occult phenomena by the psychic theory alone ; of course genuine physical manifestations require the co-operation of some sort of energy to produce them.

Attention may be drawn to the fact that materialism is completely disproved if telepathy and clairvoyance cannot be explained by physical theories. Furthermore the same holds true for every theory which considers the world as a mechanism. It is impossible. Ostwald's " energetics " are hit just as hard by it as materialism ; also positivism and the greater part of neo-Kantianism which also claims that the world is a mechanism, or at least considers all one side of the Real as such.

If it be proved that the physical and matter do not suffice to explain the facts, we must obviously concede the existence of another factor which is non-physical, non-spatial and non-mechanical, the field of which is in the main our field, the objectivity of whose phenomena was proved. As far as I know this is one of the clearest and most indisputable arguments against the idea that all Reality is part of a mechanism, and an argument which does not require long epistemological dissertations but is directly derived from experimental facts. The opposition to this whole field of research probably has its origin here. As Virchow once said, " Facts are inconvenient," and the facts are all the more inconvenient because they strike at the root of things.

TELEPATHY AND CLAIRVOYANCE

I am of the opinion that the facts of telepathy and clairvoyance shed new light on the old philosophical problem of how we are to conceive the inter-relation of body and mind. It is quite unthinkable that changes in the brain should accompany the mental process of clairvoyance, which everything leads us to believe is connected with the place of the object under consideration in some way ; for how should processes in the brain run parallel with these mental processes which are not tied down to the brain ? The case of telepathy is similar and the same argument holds good there too.

It would lead us too far to discuss the importance of this field of research for all departments of philosophy, natural philosophy, epistemology, psychology, and metaphysics ; it is clear that it must have an enormous influence on them. We have alluded to this on several occasions. But its influence is not restricted to these. It extends, further, to the philosophy of religion and to ethics ; to both of these the question of how " spirit communes with spirit " is of no little significance. If we reflect on this matter we cannot fail to realize how very important and how revolutionizing the solution of these problems would be.

Medicine also, which is still bound to a great extent by mechanical materialistic views, will be much influenced ; especially neurology and psychiatry which will be enriched by new points of view. It is to be hoped that since this field cannot be ignored any longer, investigators will set to work to sift the grain from the chaff and lop off the growths which have thriven on an uncritical occultism. It is due to the fact that science has ignored or rejected and opposed this field of research that superstitious occultism and spiritualism have grown to such an extent and taken hold of so many minds. Science must realize that it cannot succeed in its endeavours by these methods, and that it drives people who have a desire for knowledge of these things

CONCLUSION

into the hands of the mystical occultists. This reaction can be checked only when we reach and recognize the true kernel of occultism and carefully sift and classify the actual, the probable, and the possible from the outgrowths of an unhealthy fantasy. If this is not done soon it is to be feared that all who wish to know more about such matters will go for their information to those who accept the facts—to the uncritical spiritualists.[1]

Natural scientists will have much to say against the above psychical theory : they will urge that it is a convenient *asylum ignorantiæ* which can be easily rigged up in the realm of pure thought to fulfil all our wishes, just as we can imagine fairy castles with tables which lay themselves, and the like. I fully realize that we should receive more consideration if we remained on the ground of natural science. But we must give up this advantage for weighty epistemological reasons, which are generally neglected by scientists, or they would realize that purely mechanistic or " energetic " considerations are one-sided and cannot do justice to the inherent peculiarities of the psychical. This argument, and the results of the analysis of the observed phenomena, force us to consider the psychical

---

[1] It is to be feared that science may not succeed in doing this if it keeps on its pseudo-material blinkers. How many scientists have already given up the purely empirical and phenomenological way of looking at things ? The reality at the back of the phenomena is often much more intricate and living than the shell which we succeed in extracting and polishing by the scientific treatment of the question. (Cf. the law of symbolism in *Metapsychica Moderna*, Dr. William Mackenzie, 1923.) This may also be the case with the spiritualistic views and interpretations ; they, too, may sometimes be symbolic, sometimes approximations to the facts ; facts perhaps more intricate and not logically divisible, facts which, as Tischner says, are mental and not ruled by space and time. Should we not then logically rather try to get to know them by analogies, differences, and symbolisms than try to reduce them to our material or " energetic " conceptions. As Tischner points out, it is then probable that many of them are at least partly (which is the same as saying essentially) irrational, i.e. inconceivable to our corporeal brain. [*Trans.*]

in itself and to conclude that it plays the major part in the phenomena under consideration. I believe that I have succeeded in showing that the physical theories do not explain the facts and that there are, moreover, *fundamental* objections against accepting these explanations. It is the duty of the open-minded scientist to consider the possibility of other explanations, as these have failed. As far as I can see, there are no fundamental difficulties against the psychical theory ; but we see that we soon reach the limit of our power of conception. This view can only be called " mystic " if we think that the psychical itself is mystical. But as the propounder of such an accusation probably has thoughts, conceptions, etc., himself, I shall find myself in good company.

It is perhaps wise to mention that our attempt to explain telepathy and clairvoyance by a psychical theory and to assume the existence of a super-individual mind have nothing to do with spiritualism. It is often supposed that persons who accept the facts of occultism, such as telepathy and clairvoyance, are to be identified with spiritualists. But it is essential to draw distinctions here. The fact that we have been led to experience telepathy and clairvoyance and to assume the existence of a purely mental factor to explain them, which has made the existence of a super-individual mind probable, does not prove anything about the fate of the individual soul. My investigations on telepathy and clairvoyance give me no information on the subject. The question whether the individual mind continues to exist or dissolves into the mass of the super-individual mind like a drop in the ocean is a question which is not yet solved ; the propositions of spiritualism seem to me still unproven.

It is quite natural, when we consider the experimental evidence, that a purely mechanistic science and psychology should here discern an enemy which can

CONCLUSION

beat it with its own weapons—exact experiments—and, moreover, an enemy much more formidable than the purely theoretical considerations of idealistic philosophy. Idealistic philosophy seems not to have observed the advantage of joining forces with such an ally and to be rather ashamed of making common cause with those who are pooh-poohed as " mystical ".

The facts are untouched by the theoretical views we adopt. All the positivist, materialist, " energetic," and monistic philosophical tendencies deny the existence of the psychical ; either they try to explain it as a modification of matter or of energy, or they regard it as a way of treating the same reality.

But for the present this is a secondary consideration. At any rate they will have to accept the facts and try to classify them in some way in the positive sense, even if they have no theory to account for them. It should be possible to accept facts even without a theory. I fancy that " the crack in the foundation of our views on natural science " is now visible. Will science go to work to repair it and to modify the whole edifice to fit the altered conditions ?

Schopenhauer once said : " The phenomena under consideration are incomparably the most important among all the facts presented to us by the whole of experience from a philosophical point of view ; so it is the duty of every man of science to get acquainted with them and to study them thoroughly."

It seems to me that this statement has lost none of its force ; and it is to be hoped that philosophy will at last realize the significance of this branch of research.

Printed and bound by CPI Group (UK) Ltd, Croydon, CR0 4YY

01/11/2024

01782632-0010